CAREGIVERS, TRAUMA AND THE ROAD TO RESILIENCY

You Are Not Alone

By

Susan Cooney, Ph.D.

ISBN: 1-4107-4633-X (e-book)
ISBN: 1-4107-4635-6 (Paperback)
ISBN: 1-4107-4634-8 (Dust Jacket)

Library Of Congress Control Number: 2003093584

This book is printed on acid free paper.

Printed in the United States of America
Bloomington, IN

1stBooks – rev. 06/24/03

This book is dedicated to my family for their love and support and their remarkable examples of caregiving and resiliency.

Abstract

TRAUMA AND RESILIENCY IN PROFESSIONAL AND FAMILIAL CAREGIVERS

Susan P. Cooney

Previous research on trauma has shown that caregivers are not immune to secondary traumatization, burnout and the pursuant difficulties. This study investigated the residual effects of secondary traumatization on caregivers. The study explored the key factors in resiliency traits of professional and familial caregivers. Resiliency referred to the ability to rebound and adapt to difficult life events; a state of hardiness. The term "caregiver" included members of the family system or any professional engaged in the care of a victim of disability following a traumatic episode for a minimum of four years.

Participants were 20 each of professional and familial caregivers and 20 control subjects. Eight caregivers also participated in an in-depth qualitative interview. Participants were recruited through volunteer posters placed in Massachusetts and New York area hospitals

Two quantitative self-report questionaires, the Modified PTSD Symptom Scale and the Resiliency Scale and a qualitative semi-structured interview and questionaire were used. The primary variables were PTSD, resiliency, and caregiver type

The quantitative hypotheses for this study were basically confirmed; 1. There will be significant differences on PTSD scores in familial and professional caregivers compared to control participants consistent with secondary traumatization. 2. There is an inverse relationship, between the two measures of resiliency and PTSD. 3. There will be gender effects on familial and professional caregivers PTSD scores. The quantitative testing methods were; analysis of variance and Pearson Correlations.

Research questions for qualitative in-depth interview further revealed: (1) That the caretaking experience includes features of secondary traumatization and somewhat different difficulties for familial and professional caregivers of this experience; (2) Risk factors that aggravate, or protective factors that ameliorate the difficulties of the caretaking experience; (3) The value of spirituality and hope in resiliency for familial caregivers particularly; and finally,

(4) Recommendations from professional and familial caregivers to others to help them remain resilient and sustain the caregiving battle. The qualitative research questions revealed protective factors that are related to resiliency; social connectedness, self-esteem and spirituality. The implications of this study support further examination of the relationship between caregiver strain following a traumatic event and factors contributing to resiliency.

Table of Contents

Appendixes

Tables

Figures

Chapter 1

Introduction

<u>The Problem</u>

This study examines the key factors in resiliency or coping capacities, of caregivers following a traumatic episode: Why can some caregivers cope while others are unable to sustain the caregiving effort? What impact do gender and cultural issues have upon resiliency? What are the contributing factors distinguishing professional versus familial caregiving? And finally, does professional distance provide more effective care and efficacy or does increased empathy and love from a family perspective enhance and support caregivers throughout their ordeal?

What are the key factors that make some people more adaptive to trauma and vicarious traumatization than others? "Patients move on with varying degrees of functional ability, some with determination and buoyancy, others with little confidence that life is actually worth living" (Fine, 1990).

One possible response for serious illness could be fear. Is the flight or fear response in management of trauma guided by the unique makeup of a person, a case of habituation, professional distance, cognition, or a learned adaptive behavior? What are the ethical boundaries for caregivers? How do they find a balance between care for others and for themselves? One danger is that they will not respect their own needs, because their own suffering and challenges are not well understood or made allowance for.

The term "caregiver" includes members of the family system or any professional person engaged in the care of a victim of disability following a traumatic episode for a minimum of four years. Ideally, caregiving is a selfless act done for a number of reasons that may include duty, a sense of love, or compassion, or it may be based on ego, need to be needed, or social approval. However, evidence shows that caregivers have a direct reaction to the concerns and traumas of their charges. The results of this study discovered a negative correlation between resiliency and PTSD scores. There were minimal effects on PTSD symptoms based on gender, except for a small increase in symptoms for professional females.

Also, discovered are a wide array of protective factors that may be relevant, such as the level of social support and caregiver recomendations. The effects of secondary traumatization are far reaching, affecting both the familial and the professional involved in alleviating the suffering of others. Secondary traumatic stress is defined as "The natural consequent behaviors and emotions resulting from knowledge about a traumatizing event experienced by a significant other. It is the stress resulting from helping or wanting to help a traumatized or suffering person" (Stamm, 1999, p.68). Secondary trauma or compassion fatigue is a relatively new and unchartered area for the human sciences. The symptoms of burnout observed among some caregivers of distressed, disabled, or traumatized individuals are similar and seem to correspond to the symptoms of posttraumatic stress disorder (PTSD). Caregivers describe a weariness from dealing with fear and suffering on the human level during the course of everyday business. The DSM-IV calls this condition Secondary Traumatic Stress Disorder (STSD). The victims of PTSD can reach out to colleagues and family to express their overwhelmed feelings and to prevent fatigue and burnout.

Likewise, vulnerable caretakers must have the ability to calm themselves and remain connected to others as well as maintain a focus on the rewards of the task at hand.

In order to explore these issues, this study focuses on "resliency." Resiliency or hardiness is the ability to "bounce back" from adversity. "Resiliency has been conceptualized as an aggregate of specific psychosocial resources, namely ego strength, social intimacy, and resoucefulness, that promote coping efficacy" (Kadner, 1989). It is impressive to observe the capacity of people to put their own needs aside for others in a time of crisis, illness, or disability.

Another major factor in resiliency can be spirituality within the family system. After a catastrophe, some people rely on their spiritual inclinations. Hope and the ability to believe that things will get better is vital to resiliency. The adaptation of the family to serious chronic illness or trauma can create a questionable future for the family system, but the ability to hope can be a sustaining quality.

At some time in most people's lives, the difficulty of medical decision-making, loss and grief will be encountered. A clear understanding of hardiness and resiliency factors, may help to sustain strength and equalibrium through these difficult times. The exploratory hypothesis of this study is that a sense of social connectedness and understanding of personal resources, a sense of self and competency, mastery, and self-confidence are worth studying as factors that would allow us to cope. Also, a belief in spiritual meaning within an event and a flexibility to adapt to new roles with clear boundaries provides us with the necessary resources to endure an either brief or chronic period following trauma.

Statement of Purpose

The purpose of this dissertation is to analyze the emotional response of familial and professional caregivers to trauma. Secondarily, the study will elucidate key factors in resiliency. The third purpose is to study if caregivers exhibit secondary traumatization from caregiving roles after 4 years? Also, this study will addresss protective factors related to resiliency, social connectedness, gender, self-esteem and spirituality. We will examine the history of the study of trauma over the last 120 years and the recent developments of research instruments to study the emotional toll on trauma victims.

The exposure to the effects of trauma on a patient, can result in a lack of control in the caregiver's life. This outcome is measured by the frequency of the symptoms of PTSD and Acute Stress Disorder for a significant percentage of caregivers. People who develop PTSD become fixated and stuck on the trauma. Secondary Traumatization can involve caregivers to people who are victims of trauma (Stamm, Beth, 1999). These caregivers include family members, doctors, nurses, fire fighters, police officers, families, etc. This is a relatively new area of study. The research investigates the key factors that play important roles in making some people adaptive and able to rise above adversity under the same circumstances in which others suffer pathological consequences. "Personal perceptions and responses to stressful life events are crucial elements of survival, recovery, and rehabilitation, often transcending the reality of the situation or the intervention of others" (Fine,1991).

The various ways people cope and are able to endure following a trauma have commonalities in symptoms and levels of functioning.

Sometimes people go through the stages of grief, shock, searching, disorganization, and reorganization rapidly. At other times, they become stuck in one stage. At still other times, their lack of resiliency and endurance turn into a very deep and long-lasting depression. This research discusses the biopsychosocial aspects of grieving and the impact of trauma and the psychological impact upon caregivers and families following traumatic episodes.

Direct exposure to the trauma puts the caregiver at risk for secondary traumatization. The manifestations of this condition can be similar to the symptoms of PTSD.

The process of tending for a family member following a sudden trauma or prolonged or chronic illness can be exhausting. The combination of emotional vulnerability and the neglect of one's personal needs over time can be cumulatively injurious. Eventually, the caregiver can become a secondary victim of the trauma. Empathy for the patient often mutes the needs of the tending party and usurps their identity. Nancy Reagan wrote about the effects of caregiving for a loved one in her book, *I Love You, Ronnie*, (1999):

There is a feeling of loneliness when you're in this situation. Not that your friends aren't supportive of you; they are. But no one can really know what it's like unless they've traveled this path—and there are many right now traveling the same path I am. You know that it's a progressive disease and that there's no place to go but down, no light at the end of the tunnel. You get tired and frustrated, because you have no control and you feel helpless. When it comes right down to it you are in it alone. Each day is different, and you get up, put one foot in front of the other and go—and love. (Reagan, 1999, p. 184).

The symptomatology of PTSD can be observed in victims of secondary traumatization and diagnosed after three months of concurrent symptoms. The three main symptoms are intrusion, avoidance, and hypervigilance or hyperarousal. The patient feels helpless and unable to perform daily functions for fear of threatened or imagined death or injury. This study looks for symptoms suggestive of PTSD among the family caregivers. The PTSD Symptom Scale by Van Der Kolk (1995) is designed specifically to test this and is be administered as part of this study (Appendix F). As David Baldwin stated, "Traumatic experiences shake the foundations of our beliefs about safety and shatter our assumptions of trust" (Baldwin, 1997). Reactions to trauma are meant to be positive and are meant to be adaptive, but more often than not, the symptoms are instead maladaptive.

There is no clear evidence that any particular ethnicity, minority group, or gender is more prone to trauma reactions. It is a state of a person being violated, often by someone on whom they depended and having their trust broken, feeling helpless, vulnerable and/or threatened with death (Yehuda, et al., 1997).

"The coping behavior that is most frequently identified, is around the need for families to know more information about an illness, maintain control in the situation, feel hopeful and receive support" (Koller,1992, p.339).

Koller suggests that one of the most successful coping strategies during illness is to have a confrontative style that consists of addressing the problem realistically. It includes trying to get a sense of the disease, understand it, uncover information regarding different treatment programs available, thereby gaining a mastery over the illness.

Effective methods have been undertaken to protect caregivers from the risks of psychological burnout or traumatization. This study discusses the research in this area. One example is a longitudinal study that was done on traumatic injury that follows the family members' rating of coping. The effects of trauma and caregiving permeate the lives of everyone at some time during their lives. Remarkably, it is during this critical and fragile point of trauma that human beings can be their most noble.

An issue in resiliency of the family system is collaboration. This occurs when the entire family takes on the burden and responsibility of caregiving for an ill member. This is contrasted to the situation in which there are single caregivers, who can become exhausted and at times resentful, because they set aside their own needs and are unfulfilled in their own dreams. Finding the family's key resources, assessing this dynamic system, and putting together a plan is vital (Kiser, Ostoja, & Pruitt, 1988). Determining who does what to mediate the responsibility will help to develop a sense of networking and communication in the hardiness of the caregivers.

When family members encourage each other to communicate, a postive outcome will result. Each individual family member perceives events differently. The interpretation of the reactions of each member helps to validate the feelings of the caregivers. However, the ability

of each member to be flexible and understanding aids in assimilating

experiences and moving forward. In an effort to help future families

in crisis, science can help teach us how to establish protective factors

that act as a buffer and provide a context for clear thinking during

crisis. McCubbin and McCubbin state, "Families are resistant to

disruption in the face of change, and adaptive in the face of crisis

situations" (1988, p.247).

A great many people with early difficulty do not thrive. The

important question is to find what makes the difference? What

intervening or third factors may further a resilient outcome or a

creative coping and survival strategy.

> Personal and family supports and advocates, role models, high
> inteligence and other individual characteristics, personal
> opportunities, and other advantages may all contribute to
> psychological "immunization" (Richards, 1999, p.41).

Reaction to devastating events that have shattered the belief

system and trust of human beings can produce similar symptoms in

the primary victim of trauma, and in caregivers as the secondary

victims. Therefore, commonalities of traumatic response and grief may be consistent for the primary and the secondary victims of trauma. The frequent symptoms of disassociation, somatization, and affect dysregulation are prevalent in many case studies.

The impairment of affect regulation creates a tendency on the part of victims to respond appropriately to an event by over or under-reacting. An example of overeacting may be symptoms that result in insomnia and exaggerated anger, restlessness and hyperarousal.

Some of the key issues in the symptomatology of trauma, are the victim's memory distortions, dissociation, intrusive memories, and the fight-or-flight response to danger. Aggression can result from traumatic injury for some individuals, because the patient is unable to articulate what is causing so much pain and this can be incredibly frustrating. Additionally, the distress can have an impact upon the patient's relationships, whether intimate, platonic, or familial. Trauma can create a feeling of being unable to trust and and the certainty that letting down one's guard in any manner will result in further traumatization.

Unfortunately, when a patient is unable to articulate what they are feeling, the body can then manifest symptoms such as stomachaches, headaches, backaches, that are not originated as organic or biological problems. These symptoms are more a response to the psychological distress or somatization of the patient.

Background

Historical/Theoretical Perspective

The study of trauma has been ongoing for 120 years. Pierre Janet's work at Salpetriere began the field in his evaluation of hysteria. In 1889, Janet wrote about the relationship between trauma and memory:

> It has been widely accepted what is now called declarative active and constructive process. What a person remembers depends on existing mental schema; once an event or a particular bit of information is integrated into existing mental schemas it will no longer be available as a separate, imutable entity, but it is liable to become distorted both by associated experiences, demand characteristics and the emotional state at the time of recall. (Janet, 1989)

Janet found a common theme when treating trauma patients. They all appeared to have traumatic past experience, from which they were unable to move forward and experienced symptoms such as dissociation, passivity, psychosomatic complaints, and affect deregulation. Janet states;

> The remembrance of these events absorbed a great deal of energy and played a part in the persistent weakening. It failed to regulate emotional reactions to reminders of past trauma that caused some hysterics to continue to disassociate and to react with automatic, excessive and irrelevant responses. (Janet, 1996)

Hysteria was later dismissed from the psychiatric nomenclature and replaced with other diagnosis that were more specific, including Post Traumatic Stress Disorder, Somatization, Dissociative Identity Disorder, and other Axis 1 and II diagnoses from the DSM-IV.

Freud agreed with Janet when he made a visit to Salpetiere in 1880 and felt that dissociation was also;

"...the splitting of consciousness which is so present to a rudimentary degree in every hysteria. It is the basic phenomenon of this neurosis" (Freud,1896). Freud said, "After severe shock the dream life continually takes the patient back to the situation of his disaster from which he awakens with a renewed terror. The patient has undergone a physical fixation to the trauma" (Freud, 1959).

Janet and Freud further postulated that patients were so fixated on keeping their emergency response system ready for the next impending trauma that they were unable to keep their everyday life on course because they were too distracted and derailed by the prospect. Janet felt that memories of trauma were so difficult to integrate into one's schema that the memories manifested in anxiety, hypervigilence, and hyperarousal that were disassociated from consciousness (Van Der Kolk, 1994). These results disclosed significant differences between the ways people experience memories versus traumatic memories.

Another theorist who was interested in the study of trauma and how it relates to an individual's ability to move forward is William James. He stated;

> The past studies have revealed to us whole systems of underground life, in the shape of memories of a painful sort which lead to a parasitic existence, buried outside the primary fields of consciousness, and making eruptions there unto with hallucinations, pain, convulsions, paralysis of feeling and of motion, and the whole procesion of symptoms of hysteric disease of body and of mind(James in Nemiah, 1995, p. 230).

In the 1940s Kardiner (1941), studied trauma and neurosis during wartime. He formulated the diagnosis of PTSD. He stated, "The nucleus of this neurosis is a psychoneurosis. It outlives every accommodative device and the traumatic syndrome is ever present and unchanged" (Kardiner, 1935).

Also, during World War II, one of the most notable women in the evaluation and study of trauma response was Anna Freud. She conducted studies on the reaction of children to the London Blitz.

A forerunners of trauma research today, is Van Der Kolk, at the Human Resource Institute Trauma Center in Boston, Massachusetts. This study reviews some of his work and the development of trauma research instruments. They have changed the ability to evaluate patient reactions and maladaptions to traumatic events. The validity of previous research studies in human science have been compromised by dealing with non-empirical qualitative studies. However, Van Der Kolk has found a way to collate the new data analysis and evaluation of emotional experiences by using quantitative studies to further understand the inner psyche of victims of trauma. He conducted a research study and collected information that yielded a useful database for professionals and formulated the development of a field trial for PTSD criteria for the DSM-IV.

Van Der Kolk defines declarative memory to be a process that helps us integrate trauma into our mental schema. Once it has been integrated, it is no longer an individual component. The retrieval aspect influences the current state of a trauma patient when they are relooking at the past. However, when a patient has PTSD, the traumatic memory remains on a different accessible level and has stood frozen in time. The memory is not being processed or integrated into their schema. The result is memory disturbances in which the patient is unable to retrieve the memories in a clear, undistorted way. However, the actual trauma itself does not get distorted but remains fixed in time. The trauma patient generally has an uncanny ability to recall even the minutest detail of the traumatic event.

A primary or secondary trauma victim's response to even the most minor stress can be overexaggerated because of the victim's readiness to go into overdrive mode. When a people are under stress, they change their biological makeup and secrete a higher level of endogenous stress hormones that affects their memory consolidation. This in turn affects their ability exercise proper judgment in the face of incoming possible trauma, which ironically may be just a minor event.

> "The limbic system is part of the central nervous system that maintains and guides the emotional behavior necessary for self-preservation and survival of the species. It is critically involved in the storage and retrieval of memories" (Van Der Kolk,1994).

The subjects in Van Der Kolk's(1994)study, demonstrated that the memories of the trauma were recalled in fragmented pieces over time. Initially there were visual images or somatic sensations until they were put together. The conclusion was that when a person experiences an event, they consolidate it into sensory information and only integrate it into a narrative form when their conscious is aware of the memory. Initially, when a person experiences a traumatic event there may only be sensation and feeling. There is not a narrative form and this is only forthcoming over a period of time. This obvious limitation is significant and goes to the very core of the pathology of PTSD.

Weiss (1998) discusses ways to recover from the psychological impact of chronic illness or sudden trauma on families and caregivers:

Four processes seem to be required for recovery to occur. There must be cognitive acceptance of the loss. Ordinarily, this means there must be an account that provides the surviving spouse with a satisfactory explanation of how the loss came about. There must be emotional acceptance of the loss, through the mechanisms of apparently obsessive reviewing of memories and thoughts, until they are, for the most part, emotionally neutralized, and so can be lived with. There must be identity change, so that the individual understands himself or herself for that reference to the spouse, and new social linkages must be established which support the new identity (p.75).

The theorists over the last 120 years began when Janet studied hysteria which Sigmund Freud did further work describing traumatic response as dissociation and declaritive memory. Piaget followed with his exploration of integrated memory and lack of accomodation of traumatic recollection. Dr. A. Kardner and Anna Freud studied the trauma of war and found the same commonalities in response as their predecessors. Dr. Van Der Kolk is Piagetian who investigates biological responses to trauma as well as designing standardized tests with high reliability and validity to test emotional reaction to trauma. A colleague of Van Der Kolk, Dr. Weiss at the University of Massachusetts, investigates the protective risk factors to prepare for trauma. These theorists conclusions fit with one another and overlap with universal findings. Primary and secondary trauma response is a physiological and emotional reaction, that may be symptomatic of dissociation, numbing, affect dysregulation, scarring and fixation on the trauma. Therefore, this study will continue from the work of these theorists and examine the professional and familial caregiver's emotional response and potential for secondary traumatization and thier resiliency factors.

Background of the Etiology of Primary and Secondary Trauma

As far back as 1889, Pierre Janet stated that reaction to trauma had a biological base. Therefore, the significance of the limbic system in emotional reaction is key to learning to negotiate and understand the psychodyanmics of trauma. The psychobiology of trauma is related to the response of the limbic system in overdrive and is clearly a physiological phenomenon. The trauma worker helping a traumatized family is trying to help them form filters to distinguish between threatening and non-threatening stimuli.

The biological impact of trauma is observable by several methods including brain imaging. LeDoux (1996) argues that brain imaging can show lesions on the amygdula from trauma or secondary trauma. This emotional component is not simply "hysteria," as in Freud's terms, but can cause a physical injury and should to be treated accordingly. In effect, emotional trauma and its' sequellae do have a physical basis as MRI scans show. The brain has the ability to retrieve, integrate, and store traumatic memories over a lifetime.

Le Doux did many studies on the amygdala to produce conditioned fear responses and discovered that cortical lesions prevent their extinction. This led him to conclude that;

> "…once formed, the self cortical traces of the conditioned fear responses are indelible and that emotional memory may be forever" (1992).

Therefore, the responses or memories may affect the patient indefinitely, through nightmares or visual hallucinations and other symptoms of trauma. Le Doux believed that the emotional scarring and lessions on the brain developed specifically from the trauma. He supports his conclusion with pre-post traumatic MRI's.

The physiological response to secondary trauma was delineated by Seyle in 1978 and has been known as the general adaptation syndrome. This describes the hormonal response of the catecholamines and the corticosteroids, which react when the body goes into either flight and anger response or a flight and fear response. At this time, the patient cannot learn or concentrate and when there is no emotional or mental input then the patient regresses to the traumatized state.

Kolb has done many studies on excessive stimulation of the central nervous system and has shown through studies that the neuronal changes in a patient are significant and that the hippocampus exhibits lesions that are directly correlated to traumatic response. He has named this the Acoustic Saddle Response (ASR), which has characteristics of hormonal responses from intense stimuli. Kolb states,

> "Thus, the inability for PTSD to properly integrate memories of the trauma, and instead continuous reliving of the past, this merits physiologically in the misinterpretation of anocuous stimuli, such as the ASR, as potential threats" (Kolb, 1987).

Initially, this hormonal response can be looked upon as something positive to help a person deal with the incoming trauma and to allocate energy and resources for coping. However, studies have shown that over long periods of time, the emergency physiological system of a person can desensitize and not be as available when it is needed. This has been further demonstrated in research by (Davis,

1993) on neuro-endocrine abnormalities in patients who have had a trauma in the past. This process showned an impact on catecholamines, corticosteroids, serotonin levels, and endogenous opioids, which all presented levels that were significantly outside of the normal range.

> "The brain changes with experience, all experiences good and bad, and the brain changes by storing elements of a traumatic experience and allowing the individual to sense the external and internal environment, process this information, perceive and store elements of these sensations, interact to promote survival, and optimize our chances for successful mating, the key to the survival of the species. (Perry, 1999)

Ergo, if one of the major reasons for the functions of the brain is to protect a person, then it will go into overstimulation and exert every effort to provide protection from a perceived incoming threat.

The symptoms of secondary trauma that result from caregiving can be insidious and pervasive. Therapy and recently psychopharmacologic interventions can provide a way back to the victim's former level of functioning. There have been a number of attempts at psycho-pharmacological treatment of primary and secondary traumatization. These drug trials have been done with monoamine oxidase inhibitors (MAOIs), tricyclic anti-depressants, and anxiolytics as well. There is evidence of the success of selective serotonin reuptake inhibitors (SSRIs) in treating Major Depression. Paxil™, which is an antidepressant, has also proven to be helpful in the reduction of panic symptoms. One promising new medication is Fluoxetine™, the effectiveness of which provides even more evidence that PTSDs are largely related to the serotonergic system in the body. There are new drug trials and research being done all the time to seek aid for victims of primary and secondary trauma.

Unfortunately, the victims often self-medicate with illegal drugs or liquor in an effort to block the memory of the acute episode. If we are able to foster protective factors for caregivers of trauma then we can avoid these interventions.

The hyperarousal response can be experienced not only by the initial victim of trauma but by the secondary trauma victim as well. Hyperarousal is a symptom of PTSD and is characterized by a dissociative state. "The challenge is to study the arousal reaction of trauma victims and see if there is a way to reset the startle response" (Van Der Kolk,1999).

The limbic system is the part of the brain that sorts out emotions to discern which are valued and nonvalued stimuli; it adjusts the sense of feeling and the sense of relationships that are safe, whereas the amygdula is said to interpret more of the oncoming threats. Therefore, the biological reaction for the victim of trauma is similar to the response of the caregiver and family involved with the patient.

Objectives and Goals

The objectives of this dissertation proposal are to explore the effects of trauma and associated stress responses on those who work in a professional and familial caregiver capacity. Also, this study will explore the potential effects of secondary traumatization on these caregivers. The researcher will use quantitative instruments to test the participants to observe whether they exhibit symptoms of PTSD. The participants will be interviewed to determine which qualities generate resiliency. The study will address the possibility of different responses to caregiving for professional versus familial caregivers. Is "emotional distance" a factor in resiliency for professional caregivers? Finally, our qualitative instruments will focus on which methods have been helpful for the caregivers and their recommendations for others.

Hypothesis

The quantitative hypotheses for this study are;

(1) There will be significant differences on PTSD scores in familial and professional caregivers compared to control participants consistent with secondary traumatization.

(2) There is an inverse relationship, between the two measures of resiliency and PTSD.

(3) There will be gender effects on familial and professional caregiver PTSD scores.

My qualitative research questions are;

(1) What are the experiences of secondary traumatization on familial and professional caregivers?

(2) What are the protective and risk factors affecting resiliency and how do they help caregivers cope?

(3) Is gender an issue in caregiving roles and adaption?

(4) What part does spirituality and hope play in resiliency for caregivers?

There is an expectation that women will assume the caregiver role automatically without complaint is an added burden. Guilt can often ensue if a female caregiver is unable to continue with her duties; this guilt may possibly make her more vulnerable to Secondary Traumatic Stress Disorder. The presumption that a women will be tireless and nurturing is socialized from a young age. "Females' traditional socialization is into affective, nurturant-supportive, dependent and 'maternal' types of roles" (Seelbach,1977). Therefore, we will hypothsize that gender issues are an important element in the study of caregiver trauma and coping.

This study reviews research that has provided very incisive examples of the capacity for love, compassion, and caring, and the ability to put personal needs aside for others. Caring for another and for oneself requires a very delicate balance, but the sense of honor, duty, and love within family systems and caregiving roles is remarkable. The examples of resiliency throughout this literature review and in the author's work during 13 years at the Massachusetts

General Hospital in the Emergency/Trauma Department with caregivers and families are testimony to the valor of the human spirit and the instinct for survival.

After a comprehensive review of the literature in Chapter 2, Chapter 3 provides the details of my methodology, which includes both quantitative and qualitative aspects.

Chapter 2

<u>Literature Review</u>

The literature review begins with a the definitions of trauma. The review looks at primary traumatization and how it relates to secondary traumatization from a biopsychosocial perspective. The key groups considered are familial and professional as well as gender, spousal, and children's issues. The literature review concludes with a theoretical perspective. Pierre Janet (1889) first described the central issue in trauma as dissociation, that is, memories of what has happened cannot be integrated into one's general experiential schemas and are split off from the rest of personal experience. "Physiological hyperarousal seems to be a central precondition for dissociation to occur" (Rauch, 1995). Janet first coined the diagnosis Multiple Personality Disorder, which has been replaced by Dissociative Identity Disorder (DID)in the DSM-IV. This term basically describes how traumatized people become attached and fixed in the memory. Freud stated that;

These people are unable to integrate traumatic memories, they seem to have lost their capacity to assimilate new experience as well. It is as if their personality definitely stopped at a certain point and cannot enlarge anymore by the addition or assimilation of new elements (1959).

Definitions

This section discusss the definitions of primary and secondary traumatization, hardiness, resiliency, and family caregivers. The literature describes various traits of primary and secondary trauma and illustrates universal symptoms. "When a person's world is shattered by the unthinkable, terrifying experiences that rupture people's sense of predictability and invulnerability can profoundly alter the ways that they subsequently deal with their emotions and with their environment" (Van Der Kolk, 1995).

This section delineates meanings, commonalities, and definitions. As stated earlier, primary trauma is defined as "…the state of a person being violated, often by someone on whom they depended and having their trust broken, feeling helpless, vulnerable, disabled or threatened with death" (Yehuda, et al., 1997).

(1) *Secondary traumatic stress* is defined as "The natural consequent behaviors and emotions resulting from knowledge about a traumatizing event experienced by a significant other. It is the stress resulting from helping or wanting to help a traumatized or suffering person" (Stamm, 1999, p.68). Although not all caregivers develop pathological outcomes, a significant number acquire symptoms of PTSD. There are multiple names for secondary traumatization, such as Compassion Fatigue and Vicarious Traumatization, and these conditions often produce PTSD-like symptoms. Burnout is not limited to professionals in the medical field. For example, sometimes jurors have burnout due to pressures and stress. Primary and secondary traumatization includes anybody in the caregiving role that has had their sense of control, sense of energy, and emotional capabilities taxed to the maximum. If the symptoms impinge upon the ability to function and their ability to get on with other areas of life, then burnout is experienced.

The precursor to secondary traumatic stress syndrome is depression, which is basically an increase in pessimism, irritability, possible hypochondriases, neurovegetative signs of *depression,* inability to focus, and sleep disturbance. Caregiver self-esteem may also suffer during this period. This may sound incongruent when the caregiver is doing the "honorable and noble" thing in taking care of an injured family member. However, the basic needs of the caregiver can be muted, especially in dealing with chronic illness or when the outlook or prognosis is poor. The patient may no longer be a companion, and in this situation, the caregiver may sense that there is no end in sight, or sadly, that the only end in sight might be the death of a loved one.

(2) The definition of *resilience* in *Webster's Dictionary New World* (1993) may be pharaphrased to apply to the family system: "the property of the family system that enables it to maintain its established patterns of functioning after being challenged and confronted by risk factors." Another definition of resilience, "The family's ability to recover quickly from a misfortune, trauma, or transitional event, causing or calling for changes in the family pattern or function; buoyancy" (Hamilton, McCubbin, McCubbin, Thompson, & Allen, 1997, p.1).

McCubbin and McCubbin (1988) define *resilience in families* as "...characteristics, dimensions, and properties of families which help families to be resistant to disruption in the face of change, and adaptive in the face of crisis situations" (p.27).

(3) *Hardiness* in this context is the confidence and the ability to tolerate hardship. The mastery of coping skills is seen in an ecological and developmental context. The question is; what are the key factors that make a person, an individual, or family resilient? Are these factors innate trait or are they socially taught within the confines of the family system and community? Hardiness is construed as an ability to tolerate anxiety and a confidence to withstand difficult circumstances.

(4) *Intrusive reexperiencing* is one of the most common manifestations of a primary and secondary trauma reaction and consists of going about everyday life and being suddenly inculcated with flashback memories of the trauma, not by a nightmare, but in a fugue state, in which the events are relived in an altered state of consciousness. These episodes can consist of the entire event being replayed or just fragmentary pieces of the event. Fugue states are also

common in trauma victims for whom the memory of the trauma is simply nonexistent.

(5) Another symptom of primary and secondary trauma is atomic *hyperarousal*, a state in which victims are in a vigilant, alert stance, awaiting the next potential danger. The condition implies a lack of trust in their somatic stress reactions, which produces a hyperalert state that represents an attempt to take appropriate action for whatever danger may be forthcoming. The sufferer tends to stay in a state of hyperarousal in spite of a fairly good psychosocial adjustment.

(6) The *numbing response* is the opposite of hyperarousal. In the numbed state, "the patients are so exhausted from their aroused and alert state that they simply shut down. They are numb to any environmental stimuli. On one hand, the positive aspect is that they are not in a state of tremendous anxiety. However, the victim then suffers from a condition called anhedonia, which is the inability to take pleasure from or enjoy any aspect of things that used to give them pleasure. Their baseline becomes one of withdrawal and isolation in an effort to cope and to protect themselves from further injury. They feel hopeless and unable to picture any positive future

goals for themselves; they are unwilling or unable to explore the events of the trauma on a psychodynamic level." (Van Der Kolk, 1991, p. 202).

(7) Traumatic experience creates difficulty in the formulation of decisions because information processing is compromised. This can result in *dissociation*. Van Der Kolk (1995) postulates memories of the trauma, until they are synthesized into a person's schema, are continuously intrusive. The patient develops a phobia of the memory and is unable to integrate it into the past and is therefore stuck. The inability to translate memory into declarative memory can cause the trauma victim to split off this piece of their past. This is called dissociation.

(8) *Somatization:* "is marked by alexithymia, an inability to identify the emotional valence of physiological states......it seems reasonable to propose that psychological trauma is the common etiological factor that ties somatization and dissociation together" (Van Der Kolk et al, 1996, p. 86).

(9) The DSM-IV has offered a new classification called *Disorders of Extreme Stress Not Otherwise Specified* or DESNOS. (Van Der

Kolk, 1996.) This diagnosis is defined by symptoms of PTSD, but for a shorter period of time-less than one month.

(10) The *limbic system* is the part of the brain that is associated with the frontal lobe and the hippocampus and deals with issues related to trauma reactions and symptomatology.

(11) McCubbin and McCubbin (1993) defined *resiliency* as

> Adjustment, which involves the influence of protective factors in facilitating the family's ability and efforts to maintain its integrity, functioning, and fulfill developmental tasks in the face of risk factors. Adaptation, which involves the function of recovery factors in promoting the family's ability to bounce back and adapt to family crisis situations. (p.247).

(12) *Vicarious traumatization* can include the observation of someone being injured, tending to somebody who has undergone a trauma, and the critical injury of a family member, as well as chronic illness within the family system.

(13) *Affect Dysregulation:* is described as, "difficulty modulating anger, chronic self-destructive and suicidal behaviors, difficulty modulating sexual involvement, and impulsive and risk-taking behaviors. These are associated with an inability to use caregivers for

soothing or self regulatory behaviors." (Van Der Kolk et al, 1996, p 86).

(14) *Spirituality:* "the divine influence as an agency working in man; on inspiring or animating principle that pervades and tempers thought, feeling or action. The doctrine that reality is spiritual rather than material" (The International Webster New Encyclopedic Dictionary, 1975).

Familial Caregivers

The study of resiliency in individuals and families is central to helping people adapt to crisis and trauma and for finding the best stabilizing factors ie; social supports, self-esteem and spirituality or hope. Research has shown that the strain of caring for a trauma victim can result in secondary traumatization for the caregiver. The effects of witnessing or observing a traumatic event and the resulting aftermath can have a psychological impact on the family caregiver. This is now commonly called compassion fatigue. "Every disabled child or adult creates a family of caregivers whose assistance is depended on. Some caregivers manage the strain; others lack the resources and are at risk of physical or emotional breakdown themselves" (Pilisuk & Parks, 1988, p.436). Researchers have identified protective factors that correlate with a family's coping mechanisms (Hawley & Dehaan, 1996). Families cope with disaster in tremendously varied ways. The research and study of either predisposed or past methods of successful coping within the family unit can be a helpful tool in promoting strength and resiliency in families under stress.

> Three classes of stressors affect families and require management; daily hassles, personal and developmental life events, and cataclysmic events. Everyday hassles and strains include all of the burdens associated with family life, such as preparing meals, balancing budgets, celebrating birthdays, etc. The majority of the literature on family stress management and cataclysmic events focus on severe or chronic illness of a family member, death of a family member, family violence, natural disaster, and war. (Kiser, Ostoja, & Pruitt, 1998, p.88).

The coping paradigm within family systems has been researched for the last 10 to 15 years. It is difficult to research families under stress, because there are limited prenormative studies that present the risk factors or measure a family's ability to endure.

Family resiliency seems to be directly correlated with the level of cohesion and the level of communication within the family system. Family system therapy encourages renewed competency in families through positive regard, support, and communication. This results in effective coping strategies that empower the family to deepen their bonds and gain confidence. Although they may not be able to change the course of a medical illness or a death within the family, family members function with the confidence that they will prevail.

In the face of crisis, families can experience a lack of harmony and difficulty adjusting, and some do disintegrate. Yet, other families bounce back, adapt to the new situation, and alter their roles in an adaptive manner. The speed with which family members regain their balance is one of the key indicators of resiliency within the family system.

McCubbin, (1993) explains that the victim of a trauma within the family had a role; and following a trauma the other family members have to supplement that role to keep intact the integrity of the family. The hypothesis of the present research is that optimism among family members and frequent communication are key factors, as are self-esteem and the ability to maintain family integration.

The family schema is an integral part of maintaining harmony within the family system (McCubbin & McCubbin, 1988). The family system of values and beliefs may act as an anchor during periods of stress and provide the direction to resources that supply advocacy for the caregivers and the victim of the trauma or chronic illness. Baby-boomers are now becoming caregivers to the elderly, chronically ill, and disabled. This intergenerational family system has produced stressors on families and challenges their ability to cope.

Nobel Prize Laureate Kenzabuo Oe in his book, *The Healing Family*, talks about the challenges and the pain that his family experienced when his son was born with a brain abnormality that limited his functioning and mental development. Oe talks very candidly about how the family bounced back from adversity. The family members found a way to interpret, understand, and find meaning in this new course in their lives. He states,

> Families face life hardships and catastrophic circumstances, and even when they falter, they usually bounce back. It is this ability of the family to face life's challenges and seemingly unfair hardships and endure and recover that will continue to inspire family scholars to pursue this line of inquiry in the future. (Oe, 1995, p.10).

Seligman (1990), links this to optimism or learned optimism because even though there is a life-altering event, in the presence of hope, the serenity and trust that one will prevail remains. There is also the perception of a deeper meaning in the event even if things do not improve. The optimistic style is manifested in a hopeful attitude. This is very difficult with sudden trauma and chronic or terminal illness. However, the caregiver expects the family will sustain and regain their equilibrium. The hope is that although the patient may not survive, or in some scenarios the patient may be unable to return to their former level of functioning, the family members will prevail and eventually move past this difficult time. The family and the patient will learn to cope, to adapt, to create new roles and new boundaries, and to move forward after the initial shock and adaptation process are over.

Family organization and clear boundaries in the context of duties and relationships are key factors in resiliency. "A family's perception of a critical illness or injury is a subjective experience based on coping strategies, past experiences with illness, family traditions and the patient's former role in the family" (Reader, 1991, p.188).

Role differentiation and allocation may be subject to a complete reversal during the crisis, but the ability of the members to be flexible and adaptive and to regain rapid stabilization is crucial to their

overcoming the stress. The level of family functioning prior to a crisis

does appear to be a predictor of the ability of the family to withstand

the new onslaught of a trauma.

> The most common family level coping strategy involves role change or adjustment and task realignment, and a family's long term adaptation, successful or unsuccessful, is determined by an additional set of complex factors, such as the family's ability to adapt in the face of adversity and its ability to reorganize and reconceptualize the stressor to be consistent with its values, goals, beliefs, and life style. (Kiser, 1998, p.89)

After the diagnosis of an acute injury or chronic illness, the

emotional pain described by family members may include feeling

hurt, sad, afraid, devastated, and shocked. Often these feelings are

ignored in the crisis because the injured person is the main concern.

The adult female appears to be at the highest risk for emotional

problems because the burden of caregiving often falls primarily on

her, which can cause her to become socially isolated (Patterson,

1995).

> Coping is the behavioral component of capability; it is what individuals or families do to manage stress and restore family balance. The three coping strategies emphasized are investing in and working together as a family, taking care of personal support needs, and getting consultation about the medical condition from

professionals. In other words, coping was balanced between the needs of the family unit, the needs of the parent as an individual and the needs of the medical condition. (Patterson, 1995, p.54)

Task realignment or role changing during a period of sustained stress can be a healthy adaptation. When a family member becomes ill or is no longer present in the family unit, then that person's role and duties have to be taken over. The swiftness with which this happens is very important because the family can then regain their equilibrium and continue to function at least minimally in meeting the most basic needs (McCubbin, 1995). How the family perceives the stressful event and their immediate responses are of paramount import. The disruption of the homeostasis of the family needs to be corrected as swiftly as possible.

The key factors in resiliency, are the caregivers' responses to the stressor and their perceptions of it. Some families and caregivers adapt by finding meaning or higher purpose in the disaster. Their cognitive understanding, allows them to put a positive spin on negative circumstances and therefore to cope more effectively. Although denial may not be a beneficial coping mechanism. The family members' perceptions that they will sustain, comes from the basic knowledge that they have withstood adversity before. These past successes create an inner confidence, a social support network, a sense of family connectedness, and a shared belief in something other than themselves. This reconceptualizing of the stressor is a key factor in the ability to adapt. The definition of successful adaptation to trauma is the ability to keep intact roles and functioning and a sense of cohesion when faced with adversity. Flexibility, adaptivity, and very clear boundaries may help to maintain the fine balance that the caregivers and families must maintain when faced with a trauma.

> Resilient families arrive at coherent and positive understandings of stressors that are consistent with the family's shared world view. Developing a shared sense of family meaning to changes created by a family crisis is a difficult and demanding process, and the family's shared sense of congruency is achieved only through perseverance, patience, negotiation, understanding, and shared commitment to the family. Often, resilient families rely on strong religious beliefs that provide stability and meaning to their lives, especially in times of hardship and adversity. (Kiser, Ostoja, & Pruitt 1998, p.90)

McCubbin (1995) describes three characteristics seem to help a family to deal with a crisis: " (1) a clear understanding of the situation and a clear understanding of their role in the world; (2) deriving a purpose or meaning in the trauma; (3) thinking of the family as a team (i.e., more as a "we" collective, rather than as a collection of individuals); and (4) focusing on a sense of problem solving, coping ability, and developing or sustaining skills for finding resources that are available to support the ability to cope" (McCubbin & Thompson, 1993).

Families' collective coping strategies are also affected by their cultural background. Cultural context within the family is a variable that needs to be considered in all research.

> For example; A family schema in many Native American Indian and Hawaiian families is strongly influenced by several factors less prominent in Anglo families, including an emphasis on the group over the individual, a present-time orientation, and a heightened focus on spiritual beliefs and on the land. (Hawley & DeHaan, 1996, p.287).

This implies a collective approach to caregiving and a belief in a context greater than themselves.

There is a clearer understanding of the impact that the peripheral members of a patient's network can have on the course of treatment and progress. The literature on this topic provides;

> "...a guide to how social relationships determine adaptation and how these relationships may be influenced to allow more favorable outcomes...It has been established that the quality of

one's social relationships is a good predictor of how a person will deal with stress" (Coyne, 1990).

It is necessary for the treatment team to let the family know that even though life may never be the same again for the family unit, new levels of functioning and new roles will develop. The treatment team can advocate in the decision-making process and maximize the resources and strengths so that the family can thrive. The role of the therapist in providing intervention for a family experiencing stress is to help the members feel capable and to examine their available networks. Reviewing all the available information aids in understanding the trauma and gaining a mastery over it.

The concept of family resilience affirms the reparative potential in all families, and offers a valuable framework for research in clinical practice. By understanding key processes, clinicians can mobilize untapped resources, enabling distressed families to cope more effectively and rebound, strengthened through their mutual support and collaboration" (Walsh, 1996, p.277).

Children

Wollen and Wollen (1995) see resiliency as the capacity to bounce back following exposure to trauma by integrating the trauma into their thought process and to move on and repair oneself. They also note that positive parent/child relationships can provide a protective factor for children with secondary trauma, who have a sense of nurturance and connection. In addition, children with a positive role model relationship with a parent or close adult, are better able to handle secondary traumatization throughout their adult life. The role model of the parents and their ability to adjust or adapt during a crisis is observed by the child and usually mirrored Wollen & Wollen (p. 120). However, a question for future studies is: what makes two children in the same family cope differently? Luthar and Ziegler (1991) studied developmental psycho-pathology and resiliency factors for children dealing with crisis. This report on this longitudinal study of 13 years discusses certain defense mechanisms that protect children from future crisis such as role models, sense of competency and attachments.

Some researchers found that children seem to be able to cope with two stressors at one time but that a third can induce difficulties in functioning and coping. "Children can effectively cope with at least two risk factors simultaneously, but the presence of three or more risk factors almost always results in emotional or behavioral problems"

One may question these findings or wonder whether the quality of the stressor should be the first consideration. In this researcher's personal work experience, there have been children with multiple traumatic losses functioning and a child with one loss who was unable to cope.

One limitation in studies of children is that when a child is coping during a crisis, often it appears acutely, that they are very high functioning. However, the trajectory for them further down the road may be less clear. The trauma incident or episode could result in some later pathology or minimally, the development of some counter-productive defensive mechanisms within the child.

Once again, another factor to consider in resiliency is that the internal locus of control is a major factor in protecting children and adults from life stress in primary and secondary trauma. Barnard (1994) concludes that a strong sense of family support, is important to producing children that have a sense of resiliency. He favors the sociological nurture component with the family is the key system within which children learn to organize their ability to cope with stress.

The study by Kiser, Ostoja, and Pruitt (1998) revealed the family's impact on children and their ability to grow up into adults who have a mastery and competence over adversity and stated:

> (1)   the family meets the needs of each member such that satisfaction is an expected outcome, (2) the family offers a sense of security and provides the child with an identity as an individual and within the family unit, (3) the family provides the opportunity for a learned and adaptive response to stress by allowing the child to observe how other family members act during a stressful event, and (4) the family provides the child with the opportunity and ability to see the family in the greater context of the community. The children are aware that they are part of a larger network and understand their actions can have impact on the family as a whole (1998, p123).

Another question regarding the resiliency and adjustment of young children who have experienced trauma is the determination of when they may be at high risk for the development a psychological disorder. O'Grady and Metz (1987) asked why do some children who are faced with unstable home life, illness, or sudden trauma withstand the adversity and others do not? These researchers addressed this difficult question in a long-term study of adjustment of 109 children, aged 6 to 7 years, for a relationship to risk in infancy: Why are some of these children overwhelmed and others are thriving and going on to lead fulfilled lives? The concern is that it is hard to tell what future maladaptive mechanisms may be in place from the behavior of a child during the stressful event, because they may be slow to develop, perplexed, or off their usual patterns. The long-term process that may lead to pathology is unknown.

The goal is to have the children thrive and grow, individually and collectively, and to adapt and move forward in spite of the stressors. Developmental factors may be important as well:

> Similarly, older children who are highly stressed but nevertheless cope well, maybe those whose infancy was healthy and not marked by special biological, temperamental and family problems, who have close, supportive relationships with caregivers in their formative years, and have a solid sense of their own efficacy. (O'Grady & Met, 1987, p. 21).

A great problem for family and friends, when they attempt to discuss a primary or secondary trauma with a victim, is the tendency to minimize the trauma in an effort to help the patient hold it together. However, this creates an adverse reaction because the caregiver becomes more frustrated and much more distressed. The sufferer does not feel heard or understood. An example is telling children, "You are resilient; you'll get through it." This can actually be very damaging to the child's emotional, behavioral, cognitive, and social potential.

Studies by Perry et al, (1996) have shown that for children involved

in trauma

> One of the most important areas appears to be the availability
> of a healthy and responsive caretaker to provide some support,
> acknowledgement and nurturance for the child following the
> trauma. The presence of a healthy caretaker can diminish
> dramatically the alarm response of the dissociative young child.
> (Perry et al, 1996)

The child's ability to survive, is largely dependent on the fact that

although they have had their trust shattered, they can again sense and

develop trust through another caretaker. This can help their adaptive

responses become constructive rather than maladaptive.

It is profoundly sad for a child to be traumatized, because their

trajectory into future decades is changed entirely. The number of

domestic and childhood abuse cases are on the rise, and the scope of

the outcomes is even more devastating as the cycle of violence

continues down through the generations. "Conservative estimates of

the number of children in the United States exposed to traumatic

events in a given year exceed 4 million" (Perry, 1994).

For children, the many consequences of exposure to trauma can

include difficulty learning. Children who are developmentally impaired by trauma-related injuries can have poor concentration and can sometimes regress to the time and place of the trauma. Bowlby (1969) has performed child studies using attachment theory. He says;

> A rapidly expanding body of research has shown that disturbances of childhood attachment bonds can have long-term neuro-biological consequences. In addition to this disturbance in affect regulation, a large variety of studies both in animals and in human have shown that childhood abuse, neglect, and separation have far-reaching bio-psychosocial effects, including lasting biological changes which effect the capacity to modulate emotions, difficulty in learning new coping skills, alterations in immune competency, and impairment incapacity to engage in meaningful social affiliation. (Bowlby, 1969).

This follows our line of inquiry that traumatization can affect social connectedness, self-esteem and the childs ability to bounce back and be resilient.

Spousal Caregivers

This section discusses several factors related to spousal caregiver resliency and the power of endurance. The stresses of managing the medical treatment plan and financial concerns following trauma can cause conflict and strain on the spousal relationship. But, by focusing together on the task at hand the couple can move forward with a sense

of efficacy in accomplishing what needs to be done.

"Maintenance of structure, routine, and continuity, despite the added burden of a chronically ill member, tends to help families endure" (Kiser, Ostoja, & Pruitt, 1998, p.94).

Traumatic injury, chronic illness and pain management are serious and significant stressors. They do not have a small window of adaptation but are relentless in their continued responsibility and disruption of equilibrium within the family system.

Adaptation of families to serious, chronic, or life-threatening illness in a spouse or parent also has profound consequences for family life. When an adult family member becomes ill or incapacitated, the entire family must make adjustments to deal with the loss of that adult's contributions. (Kiser, Ostoja, & Pruitt, 1998, p.93)

It is important to reframe the expectations for the patient and caregiver after the initial diagnosis and adjustment. Instead of caregivers allowing continued disappointments to frustrate them and resentment to build, resilient spouses will change their expectations and adjust to the situation of the chronically ill partner.

"It appears crucial that both spouses and patients be adequately informed and have realistic expectations and well-defined tasks that allow them to manage their needs and to contribute to a positive outcome" (Coyne et al., 1990).

The caregiver must guard against social isolation, because that can be the beginning of a new and destructive pattern. Subsequently, the seclusion and remoteness from friends and family will not allow the caregiver to renew. Caregivers will mute their own needs, they will say, "Well, I'll get to that later" or, "There's time enough for that; this is my primary goal; this is my responsibility currently." But, for the caregivers to continue to help with chronic illness it is necessary for them to be able to sustain their own sense of confidence, self-esteem, interactions, connectedness, and optimism.

Helping spousal caregivers feel empowered is another factor in creating resiliency. The grueling schedule of a medical treatment regime can provide caregivers with a concrete method of contributing to the battle against trauma or illness. This provides the ability to fight back and allows some control over the situation. Although it may be an exhausting medical regime, it can provide a source of sustenance and strength for the caregiver.

A medical illness within the family, that is, a chronic condition or terminal illness, can create secondary problems from a spousal perspective. The ability of the caregiver to maintain connection with the other members of the family while under duress can be difficult to accomplish, because of a modification of the roles and expectations. One behavioral approach by Leske (1998) for coping with chronic illness indicates that the caregiver is much better off keeping an emotionally modulated response to the crisis rather than pretending to cope magnificently and being overly cheerful. When the caregiver can do it no longer, the result can be to resort to severe despair with resultant highs and lows. Rather then pretending to be able to cope, one recommendation is that the spousal caregiver simply be as communicative and insightful as possible. When the spouse is feeling bad, caregivers should admit to themselves or their spouse that they are feeling unhappy or overwhelmed. If the caregiver who is experiencing secondary traumatization mutes true feelings in an effort to support the patient, the result is likely to be a pendulum swing of emotions. Caregivers need to maintain some moderation in their emotional responses.

This is not to say that the spousal caregiver will avoid going through the grief stages of denial, anger, and guilt over the disappointment of some of their hopes and dreams. The ability of each family member to understand each other's ways of dealing with the trauma are crucial in the adaptation of crisis within a family system. Bio-psycho-social problems within the family system can further add to the difficulties at hand. Clear roles, boundaries and expectations are crucial in an ability to maintain hardiness and functioning.

> Successful coping depends on large part on the ability of the couple to avoid being destabilized by these pressures. However, the family is likely to be isolated from friends, relatives, and co-workers from outside the affected area, who do not share the perspectives of the victim (Edelstein, 1988, p. 117).

Professional Caregivers as Victims of Secondary Traumatization

Helping professionals, such as social workers, psychologists, psychiatrists and therapists, firefighters, police, etc., are also potential victims of secondary traumatization. Edward Messner (1993) did studies in resiliency enhancement and coping strategies for professionals who are confronted with the constant onslaught of trauma victims' dilemmas and anguish. In an effort to find a balance, Messner cautions the at-risk professionals to be aware of their altered equilibrium and "a tendency to react to stress with an excess of feeling and instead an excess of cognition" (p.46). Messner suggests that therapists can better gain control of their anger or their increasing resentments by understanding their reactions, or over-reactions to something that has happened by being aware of their personal inner dialogue. His premise of an internal dialogue helps such professionals to have a clearer perception of what they are feeling.

An imbalance of affect and cognition, such as intellectual understanding but with a labile emotional stance is better dealt with in the present. For example, the caregiver becomes numb so that feelings are not available. Messner recommends asking the question, "What am I avoiding? Is there a feeling that I am avoiding?" He is a strong advocate of fantasies, playing out even one's aggressive fantasies, in dealing with anger. One might find that a bit disturbing for some clients. But, Messner (1993) states that the acknowledgment of anger and then acting on it through visualization can be a cathartic tool. He states this can be a restabilizing force and can give therapists the buffer they need to continue in the caregiving battle.

The professional caregiver is not immune to secondary traumatization from interactions with their distraught patients. Although professional distance can go a long way in assauging the emotional impact of the patient's distress, it is not a fail-safe remedy. The caregiver's human emotional response is a definite factor in compassion fatigue or burn-out for the professional. There are limited studies in this area and more research is needed.

There is a tremendous burden connected with the basic caregiving and survival of other human beings, and this presents the dilemma for the caregiver of duty precluding choice.

> The data suggest that the level of subjective burden is not likely to be reduced through intervention measures since it is related to characteristics of the caregiver that cannot easily be altered (e.g., income and age). Second, the data suggests that interventions that free the caregiver at least temporarily would be effective in reducing the objective burden. (Montgomery, Gonyea, & Hooyman, 1985).

Often lost among the family and professional treatment team that are treating the victims of trauma are the peripheral members of the family. These members are sometimes affected to a greater degree than the patient, if the patient is in a vegetative state and getting adequate support relative to the injury. The often ignored, frightened, confused, overwhelmed family member is expected to stand by and be strong. This limited support and a lack of validation can add insult to injury.

Critical Incidence Stress Debriefing (CISD) groups are set up after disasters and violent incidents to provide support for victims and their families as well as emergency personnel who are responding to the situation. Surprisingly, research studies have shown that debriefing episodes are not helpful and longitudinal studies actually show that a slower adaptive process occurs when there have been such debriefings (Ursano, R., Fullerton, C. 1994).

The therapist's assessment of the family's needs and levels of functioning, cultural aspects, and roles is key to finding equilibrium, rebalancing, and adapting to the stressors at hand. It is important to validate each individual family member's emotional response to a trauma. When the lines of communication are kept open about individual coping styles, then misunderstandings can be avoided.

A victim of primary or secondary trauma may have a distorted view of themselves based on the shame or terror of what happened to them. Realigning this perception can be a difficult task when they are defensive and are entirely resistant to the reintegration of this event into their consciousness.

> The massive defenses that initially established emergency protective measures, gradually relax their grip upon the psyche so that the dissociated aspects of experience do not continue to intrude into one's life experience and thereby threaten to re-traumatize an already traumatized victim. (Van Der Kolk, 1995).

Another maladaptive behavior commonly used for mastering this response to trauma is to create defensive reactions to a trauma. Pavlov was successful in showing that negative threatening stimuli were capable of eliciting defense reactions in patients. Pavlov discovered that changes in temperament were directly related to defensive mechanisms such that the victim developed coping mechanisms to deal with their symptoms. Trauma allows its victims to sense their existential helplessness. They become exposed and vulnerable because their trust is destroyed and the unthinkable has happened to them. Their perception is that nothing in their life will ever be the same. This is truer than they probably know because the ripple effect of symptomatology and the scarring can be so extensive.

Theoretical Perspectives

This section discusses the challenge model, developmental, and family systems theory. Intact family systems, as well as an emotionally supportive climate are key elements in resiliency of individuals. These individuals seem to go on to choose spouses who are equally healthy and well adjusted. They have a strong social support network of aquaintances, friends, work colleagues, etc. It is extremely significant to have a healthy social network and strong relationships in the systemic view of resilience.

> An ecological perspective is required to take into account child-hood and adult spheres of influence in risk and resilience. The family, peer group, school or work settings and logical social systems can be seen as nested contexts for social competence. (Bronfenbrenner, 1990, pp. 27).

Seyle (1978) has studied the construct of adaptation to stress and resiliency and suggests that there may be different approaches. He stated that individuals need to have a sense of control, an optimistic outlook, and a responsibility for their actions. They need to have an understanding that if they work at something, the outcome will be relatively predictable. This outlook provides a sense of control and stability that may allow caregivers to feel that they are not helpless and they have some impact on the results of the trauma. Perhaps the caregiver will not be able to change the stressor, but they definitely can assist in coping with it.

The challenge model, is based on observing several clients and families who have been victimized and focusing on their resilient strengths. The family interpretation and sense of meaning in the trauma is key for the family to be able to move forward and formulate the family system re-adaption model.

Some people are born with greater timidity and anxiety and others with more curiosity and more outgoing temperament. However, in the developmental perspective, the traits of resiliency are not something with which one is born but that occur over years and through life experiences. They are subject to positive and forward movement, but are a compilation of life experiences. The various phases throughout the life cycle require different challenges. Resiliency is the concept of knowing that whatever difficulty occurs, one will be able to withstand, survive, and move forward.

The cognitive perspective, in helping individuals cope with stress, suggests that the primary goal is reduction of the levels of stress.

When the pressure is alleviated, the patient can think more clearly, thereby gaining some mastery over the situation. Unfortunately, a trauma victim is persistantly gearing up for a renewal of the trauma and is in a hypervigilant state and the slightest non-connected stimuli can throw the patient back into a flight or fear response. Therefore, people may not count on their usual emotional responses, which creates a loss of affective modulation. Difficulties with affect regulation and issues of unmodulated anger toward oneself, may result in risky, self-destructive behavior such as cutting.

Unfortunately, a victim of trauma can continue to have reactions to a traumatic experience for 30, 40, 50 years after the initial experience. As stated earlier, traumatic moments become fixed in time and are not integrated into the schema of the person. This may be so because of the significant changes in stress hormones in people diagnosed with PTSD. (Kolb, 1987).

Treatment of Secondary Traumatization of Caregivers

We have hypothesized that secondary traumatization may occur in familial and professional caregivers and that the symptoms mimick

PTSD. The following discussion of treatment attempts to further clarify and identify resiliency factors.

"The treatment of PTSD has three principle components: 1) processing and coming to terms with the horrifying, overwhelming experience, 2) controlling and mastering physiological and biological stress reactions, and 3) Re-establishing secure social connections and interpersonal efficacy" (Van der kolk & Fisler, 1995).

The premise is that the trauma victim needs to have a sense that the historical event that happened in their life has a certain place in time and is no longer a part of everyday life. They need to understand that the chance the trauma is going to re-play itself imminently is not realistic. The traumatized person must review, clarify, and reintegrate the event and re-incorporate it into their schema. There must be a sense of security and the feeling that life is stable and predictable. The belief in a safe environment will allow them to be able to work on self-regulation and moving forward. The patient's ability to tolerate emotions can dictate the different phases of re-looking at the trauma, because a secondary injury is always a possibility.

Ursano (1992) felt that trauma workers need to help people be grounded in the present and learn to re-process incoming information.

Family members or caregivers in a professional context ie; social workers, psychologists, psychiatrists and mental health workers, must go through the post-integrative process with the patient following trauma. This is important in helping a person to cope and process information and integrate it properly, so that they do not become stuck. This has to be done by keeping a very low arousal state. The new eye movement de-sensitization re-processing (EMDR) tool can tend to be too arousing, although it is often helpful. The procedure may augment the level of anxiety the trauma victim sustains and can often be damaging unless it is carefully monitored (Van Der Kolk, 1995).

Lazarus (1993) shows that the focus of the impact

of the trauma is actually related to the personal interpretation of the trauma, more than the trauma itself. Psychodynamic therapy is key for victims of primary and secondary traumatization to help them to put their feelings into words. Having a cognitive under-standing of what happened helps to minimize their injury.

The trauma can only be worked through when a secure bond is established with another empathic person and this can be utilized to hold the psyche together when the threat of physical disintegration is re-experienced. Once the traumatic experiences have been located in time and place, a person can start making distinctions between current life stresses and past trauma and decrease the impact of the trauma and their present experiences. (Van Der Kolk, 1995).

Research on Trauma

Only recently has literature on trauma included those who have been traumatized without actually experiencing the trauma first hand (Stamm, 1998). This section reviews the current literature on secondary traumatization as it relates to the spouse, children, the family system as a whole, and the professional caregivers. These studies explore the daunting challenge of resiliency, following a devastating trauma.

One of the first studies of crisis and secondary traumatization was by Lindemann in 1944 after the Coconut Grove fire in Boston. This longitudinal study of the grief reactions of friends and families of the victims, was one of the first studies to reveal that psychological crisis is often a result of a traumatic event. He stated;

"An apparent attempt to compensate for chronic hyperarousal, traumatized people seem to shut down on a behavioral level by avoiding stimuli reminiscent of the trauma; on a psychobiological level by emotional numbing which extends to trauma related in everyday experience" (Lindemann, 1944).

Pollack (1972), discussed the consistency in crisis and in responses. The Pollack study participant's consisted of 68 male and 86 female students. The subjects were asked to list in order of severity, the largest crises of either primary or secondary trauma in their lives and the subsequent reaction. Pollack states,

> Frustration accounted for more than the predicted 50% of severest crises, responsive flexibility rather then the predicted consistency was found, which has implications for personality theory. The level of frustration appears to sensitize people to perceive subsequent crises similarly when in fact, they may be different. The data suggests that psychotherapy should focus on new perceptions rather than new responses. (p. 691)

A study of primary trauma by Gottesman (1982) on the differences in crisis reactions upon cancer and surgery patients N=62, suggests that the crisis period can last up to 28 weeks after surgery. He studied routine surgery patients versus surgery patients with serious cancer, and showed the crisis levels were more intense with cancer. What this study has surmised is that crisis theory shows that psychological changes grow and go through the process of stabilization, even if the crisis itself does not get mitigated. This is part of the process of developmental PTSD. So in essence, even if the crisis itself is not resolved, the trauma victim eventually will regain his equilibrium.

A research study by Astin, Lawrence, and Foy (1993) involved battered women, PTSD, and factors connected with their resiliency. The participants were 33 battered women in a Los Angeles area shelters. They completed the PTSD symptom checklist and the Impact of Event Scale, a 15-item self-report measure.

> Multiple regression analysis revealed that violence, exposure, severity, recency of the last abuse episode, social support, inter-current life events, intrinsic religiosity, and developmental family stresses, predicted 43% of the variance in PTSD symptomatology. (p. 17).

Patterson (1995) underscores the importance of balance in maintaining equilibrium and coping with stress and trauma. She reiterates the importance of rapid stabilization so as not to create secondary problems such as developmental, emotional, or other bio-psycho-social issues for the other members of the family.

Resiliency/Hardiness Research

Research on the protective factors in trauma and resiliency has been a broad area of study. There have been numerous studies since the late 1970s regarding individual adaptation to coping with stressors. These studies (Caplin, 1964; Fink, 1995; Flannery, 1986; Gottesman & Lewis, 1982; Lewis, Gottesman, & Gutstein, 1979; Pollack, 1972) have focused on the individual traits of confidence and self-esteem that seem to be pervasive throughout high adaptation. They further elucidated that a positive demeanor and optimism, while helpful in adjustment, are actually not key factors in coping strategies.

A study by Hamburg and Killilea (1985) N=35, discussed the hypotheses for support as a major factor in resiliency. The four points they make are,

> ...social support can have a direct effect on health, it provides a buffer against effects of high stress, it has a mediating effect that stimulates the development of coping strategies or mastery, and lastly, a lack of social support exacerbates the impact of stressful life events.

The authors observed that patients who had not had good social supports were more apt to become despairing, develop medical illness, and were often suicidal.

Nolan (1992) conducted a research study n=38 regarding coping strategies for patients with organ transplants and coping and perceived stress of cardiac patients. It took place in five tertiary care centers with 38 family members of patients. The instruments consisted of family members completing self-report scales. The results showed that family members felt that;

> "Coping strategies used in order of decreasing frequency [were]; one, knowing our family has the strength to solve our problems, two, facing problems head on, and three, seeking support from friends" (p. 545).

A study by Lindsay and Hills in 1992 discussed the concept of hardiness. The researchers attempted to define the term and used the Composite Hardiness Score as a measurement scale. As previously mentioned, the definition of hardiness is described as the confidence and the ability to tolerate hardship. The mastery of coping skills is seen in an ecological and developmental context.

The question remains; what are the key factors that make a person, an individual, or family resilient? Is this an innate trait, or is it something socially taught, within the confines of the family system and community? Resiliency/hardiness are construed as an ability to tolerate anxiety and the confidence to withstand difficult circumstances. The measurement scale was a test that measured and described the attributes of hardiness. The Hardiness Scale is composed of a list of seven specific attributes that seem to predict hardiness.

> There is a curiosity to find meaning in experiences, a belief in being influential through what is imagined, and expectation that change is normal, and that they need to be flexible, a belief that change is an important stimulus to development, an element of self-assertiveness, and the ability and capability to endure. (Lindsay, 1992, p. 43)

In his study of resiliency factors, Rutter (1993) states that

> All studies of risk factors have shown a very considerable variability in how people respond to psychosocial adversity. Even with the most dreadful experiences, it is usual to find that a substantial proportion of individuals escapes serious sequeli. The reality, of course, is that no one has absolute resistance; rather, it is more appropriate to consider susceptibility to stress as a graded phenomenon. (p 626)

Holaday and Terrill (1994) conducted a study on resiliency and variables in children with severe burns. The literature review presented the opinion that resilient youngsters with primary trauma had an optimism and a belief that things would get better. This illustrates the commonalities of coping mechanisms between primary and secondary trauma. The victims of secondary traumatization appear to survive by using similar coping methods, that is, strong sense of self, a strong role model, and a sense of personal control and self-preservation. In the test performed at Shriner's Burn Institute in Texas, the researchers studied 98 severely burned patients between the ages of 6 and 21. The study participants were divided into a control and non-control group and were given the Rorschach Clinical Rating scale as well as the Coping Deficit Index(CDI). One of the biases of the sample was that the researchers knew the patient's, because most of them had been in the hospital for months. Holaday & Merrill(1994) results concluded;

> The personality characteristics targeted for growth should include a perception of personal control and independence rather than dependent helplessness or hopelessness. A stable self-esteem, positive self-regard, a sense of self-confidence, and a capacity and desire for satisfying an intimate relationships with others, rather than isolation and withdrawal, and an ability and willingness to tolerate stress with the capacity for control under most situations (p. 460).

Flannery (1994) discussed the successful response to crisis within people who anticipate that their coping mechanisms will sustain them and will grant them a mastery over whatever problem solving is necessary. These participants expectations of efficacy diminished their anxiety and depression. They had confidence and felt that the outcome of their crisis was going to be handled. Using the Locus of Control Scale and the Generalized Expectancy Success Scale, Flannery tested 84 people who had experienced primary and secondary traumatic events.

> "The Locus of Control Scale is a 28-item self-report measure which discusses the person's perceived control of their environment and their expectations regarding outcome (Flannery, 1986, p. 201).

The results were remarkable for showing no gender differences. The overall outcome showed that confidence and good problem-solving skills reduced the impact of stress during a crisis period. However, the common reaction throughout the studies on responses following trauma appears to be anxiety and depression as well as loss of self-esteem.

Caregiver Research

Recent studies on caregivers discuss the motivating factors behind caregiving. The research literature elucidates the various responses of families with a medical crisis and trauma. One of the difficulties of family coping during a chronic or critical illness is that if the family is not adaptive in their functioning they can hinder the recovery of the patient (Hamburg & Killilea, 1985). Lack of adaptivity presents not only a difficulty in terms of the caregiver's coping methods, but obviously bears directly on the ability of the patient to stabilize or recover.

A study by Silva (1987) discusses the impact of surgery on the caregiving spouses of patients. The Roy Adaptation model asked the spouses the most important thing they felt they needed during their wait for a patient during surgery. They concluded unanimously, that it was psycho-social support. Also, they needed to have a sense of control, feel they were being informed, and that their spouse was receiving appropriate care. If they were not given this information, the families' anxiety and their inability to cope increased.

In another study regarding family adaptation, Atkins & Armenta (1991) n=26, conducted the McCubbin Stress and Coping model as a framework to compare the differences in family adaptation to AIDS and other terminal illnesses. The results stated that;

When 26 families of AIDS patients and 26 families in a hospice all took the Family Inventory of Life Events and Changes Scale and the Family Adaption to Medical Stressors Questionaire, families of AIDS patients had more stress, and more rules prohibiting emotional expression and lower levels of trust then the other families. (p.71)

In another study of head injury and caregivers N=19, Mirr (1992) discussed the decision-making issues regarding life sustaining treatment. Caregivers tend to be more malleable and less decisive when they are feeling fragile and shattered by the illness of a loved one. Mirr cites four principles underlying proxy decision making: "ethical value principles, guidance principles, authority principles, and intervention principles"(p. 242).

It is important to assess the influence of the family resource because of the effect on the caregiver within the family. In her study n=107, Fink (1995) identified three types of resources in to explain strains and well-being in families providing care to an elderly patient. The key factors examined were social support, internal system resources, and the caregiver's appraisal of caregiving. Fink's study states, "Seven million American households now contain an individual who is helping an older adult with personal care or household management" (1995, p. 139). The strain of caregiving for a family member can have an impact on the well-being of the caregivers, their morale, and physical health.

Kosciulek (1997) studied the relationship of family to adaptation to brain injury n=87. His conclusion was, "An extensive and expanding body of empirical research provides firm evidence that brain injury damages families, socially, emotionally and financially" He discovered that as time went by, the size of the social network diminished, that more and more people dropped out of the picture, and therefore the caregivers were left in an isolated position to carry the strain by themselves. Again, this is where role adaptation plays a key part, because the role once assumed by the brain-injured person has to be taken on by other family members, whether it was a financial, nurturing, or other role. Anxiety and distress are present from one month to one year after the initial injury. Kosciulek's (1997) study showed that;

> "Two to six years after the injury, family members exhibit depression, drug and alcohol abuse. Finally, the report shows that family functioning is negatively affected by personality changes in the person with the injury and the day-to-day strain of meeting

the patient's needs for up to ten to fifteen years, post-injury period" (Kosciulek, 1997, p. 822).

In a recent study by Rhoades and Mcfarland of caregiver motivation, N=42 they stated;

> Quantitative and qualitative analysis yielded five categories of caregiving meaning: other directed, altruistic, self-directed, self-actualization, and existential purpose in life. Caregivers most often refer to altruistic themes. The most common one is that they do it to help others. The next most common theme was home and family duty, and the third, making a difference. (Rhoades & Mcfarland, 1999, p. 291)

This is not a simple issue. There are differing levels and variables and methods to caregiving coping strategies that are not easily defined, and therefore, make bias in research a very real difficulty.

Twibell conducted a study of family members' n=59, coping responses during critical illness suggests that;

> Family members of critically ill patients use confrontative and optimistic styles of coping most often and most effectively. Family members experience deep emotional turmoil during critical illness and need to use focused coping responses. Less healthy behavioral responses of family members during critical illness include an increased use of alcohol, cigarettes, medications, talking, eating, and sleeping poorly. Perceptions of the patient's chance of recovery were directly related to the effectiveness of optimistic, supportive, and palliative coping styles. (Twibell, 1998, p. 101)

It appears that older family members may cope better than younger family members on the average. This is explained by the fact that the older members have had more life experience. They have seen the ups and downs and vicissitudes of life and realize that more often than not, one does survive and adjust. A major coping strategy is control over one's emotions and a confidence that one will prevail. Readjusting the mental outlook and realigning expectations with reality.

A study by Leske & Jiricka (1998) discussed the impact of strengths, and capabilities on family well-being and adaptation after various critical injuries. This study examined the demands prior to the stress. Leske used the resiliency model of family stress on 51 family members within a time frame window of two days after the critical injury. Results showed that family demands are significantly related to decreases in family strength and family adaptation. This is helpful in discerning how much intervention a family is going to need and what resources and amount of assistance will help them through this crisis period. Leske and Jiricka cite an adverse relationship between increases in family demands and decrease in family strength. This is helpful information for those wishing to intervene and assist on a therapeutic level. One of the key answers to the question of helping people be adaptive and resilient following a crisis, seems to be protective factors.

Theoretical Research

There are research studies on the key concepts of coping as a theory. Interestingly, Lewis, Gottesman, and Gutstein (1979) state;

> A preliminary picture of a crisis victim shows him to be initially overwhelmed by feelings of anxiety and helplessness. In time, his inability to escape or exert control over the situation leads to despondency and a decreased sense of faith in himself. Through the first eight weeks of the crisis, these feelings become increasingly more serious. (p.132)

Caplin (1964), stated that psychological equilibrium does return within an 8-week period based on the natural healing response of the body. Gottesman (1982) states,

> The resolution of a crisis may be positive or negative, but the main point of the theory is that resolution takes place in a short time, even if the precipitating causes of the crisis are still present. [Caplin's] …premise has become a cornerstone of crisis theory, despite the fact that there is little empirical evidence to support it (Gottesman,1982, p.387).

Flannery (1986) tested n=84 consisting of 24 men and 60 women, to measure personal control as a variable on life stressors. He hypothesised that expectations of efficacy were self-fulfilling. This research as described by Flannery, involves two approaches; one emphasizes style and discusses coping as a personality trait; the other discusses it as a process and emphasizes the efforts to manage stress shaped by an adaptational context. Each of these approaches has limitations separately, but combined, they provide a unique way of studying the different adaptational processes of stress.

It appears that crises with different and variable contributing factors nevertheless have a commonality in basic reaction. One of the surprising results was that people are initially flexible and less rigid following a crisis than is commonly thought in personality theory. After the shock subsides and PTSD symptoms begin to manifest, some caregivers can become more rigid and fixed in fear of a new trauma. "Family resilience is the path a family follows as it adapts and prospers in the face of stress, both in the present and over time. Resilient families respond positively to those conditions in unique ways, depending on the context, developmental level, the interactive combination of risk and protective factors, and the family's shared outlook" (Hawley, 1996, p. 293).

<u>Summary</u>

The symptoms of primary trauma may be similar to the symptomotology of secondary traumatization and PTSD for familial and professional caregivers. A sense of confidence and self-esteem, social connectedness, spirituality, and a meaning in the experience were factors in resiliency.

The familial caregivers of victims of trauma are at risk for PTSD. Following a serious trauma in their lives, they may often be unable to understand how to respond appropriately to illness or injury to a family member. Some caregivers immediately go into a hyperaroused state, which impairs their ability think clearly (Van Der Kolk, 1994). This hyperaroused state can manifest in avoidance or in an overcompensating panic, all in an ill-conceived effort to shield themselves from the oncoming disaster. The internal world of some caregivers can be a place of fear and an alert state; they are vigilant in their effort not to perseverate and remember the injury. Yet, others function and adapt to their circumstances and even learn from the experience.

Caregivers with secondary traumatization may find that they are unable to trust their ability to discern between the proper avenue of action, or what Freud called experimental action.

"The treatment of PTSD has three principal components: 1) Processing and coming to terms with the horrifying, overwhelming experience; 2) Controlling and mastering physiological and biological stress reactions; and 3) Reestablishing secure social connections and interpersonal efficacy" (Van Der Kolk & Fisler, 1994).

The premise is that victims of secondary trauma-tization need to have a sense that the historical event that happened in their life has its own place in time and is no longer a part of their everyday life. They need to understand that the chance that the trauma is going to replay itself imminently is not realistic. The caregiver must review, clarify, and reintegrate the event and reincorporate it into the schema. The caregiver and patient need to have a sense that they are secure, that life is stable and predictable. If they feel they are in a safe environment, then they will be able to work on self-regulation and moving forward with their lives. The caregiver's ability to tolerate can dictate the different phases of relooking at the trauma, because in the absence of caution, additional injury is always a possibility.

The caregivers' self-views in light of what happened must be realigned. This can be a difficult task when they are defensive and entirely resistant to the reintegration of the event into their psyche.

> The massive defenses that initially established emergency protective measures, gradually relax their grip upon the psyche so that the dissociated aspects of experience do not continue to intrude into one's life experience and thereby threaten to re-traumatize an already traumatized victim. (Van Der Kolk & Fisler, 1995).

Primary and secondary trauma allow people to sense their existential helplessness. They become exposed and vulnerable because their trust is destroyed and the unthinkable has happened to them. Their perception is that nothing in their life will ever be the same. This may be truer than they probably know, because the ripple effect of symptomatology and the scarring can be so extensive.

Treatment implications are changing daily. However, the majority of patients are suffering far more than they let on. This is part of the symptomatology of the disease, which is to minimize or to ignore. It is poignant that the victims of secondary traumatization have forever had the security of their world shattered. Their basic assumptions in life have been challenged and the unthinkable has happened. Therefore, their trust factors will never be the same and their ability to cope will never be the same.

The efforts of the psychological communities to find relief and to understand the course and the diagnosis of PTSD will provide a respite for the caregivers. This study further elucidates the resiliency factors that help familial and professional caregivers to cope and thrive. It appears that the disturbing symptoms of compassion fatigue, burnout, and secondary traumatization are similar to those of PTSD from primary trauma. This study attempts to discover key attributes, either learned or inherent, that sustain the caregiver of the traumatically injured, chronically ill, or disabled patient.

The quantitative hypotheses for this study are;

(1) There will be significant differences in PTSD scores in familial and professional caregivers compared to control participants consistent with secondary traumatization.

(2) There is an inverse relationship, between the two measures of resiliency and PTSD.

(3) There will be gender effects on familial and professional caregivers PTSD scores.

One of the difficulties in conducting research studies on caregivers of trauma victims is the difficulty of before and after evaluations. It is difficult to assess a participant after a trauma and compare the results with the patient's pretrauma status. The coping and adaptive abilities are difficult to assess prior to the incident because we never know who is going to be the victim of a trauma. In an effort to accommodate this deficiency, some researchers have done longitudinal studies that follow the patient over a lengthy period of time until they regain some equilibrium. On occasion, post hoc assessments of patients during previous psychiatric interviews can be used and compared to follow-up evaluations after the trauma. However, this is not an ideal situation. Interpretation of retrospective data is not necessarily a reliable, ethical, or practical consideration.

Psychodynamic therapy is key to helping victims to put their feelings into words (McCann 1990). Having a cognitive understanding of what happened will help to minimize their injury.

The secondary trauma can be worked through when a secure bond is established with another empathic person and this can be utilized to hold the psyche together when the threat of physical disintegration is re-experienced. Once the traumatic experiences have been located in time and place, a person can start making distinctions between current life stresses and past trauma and decrease the impact of the trauma and their present experiences. (Van Der Kolk, 1994).

Many clinicians treat patients with psychodyanmic therapy. However, more recently, cognitive and behavioral approaches have been aimed at working with patient symptoms. The concern is that cognitive treatment is reorienting, but ignoring the past trauma may be more damaging in the long run. This treatment approach is an attempt to relieve the intrusive, affective, and somatic symptoms. A psychodynamic exploration of the past injury and trauma, in a manner that the patient can tolerate, is the best way to deal with a traumatic life experience. Van Der Kolk (2000) states,

Problems of somatization and affect dysregulation might most usefully be addressed helping patients acquire skills that help them label and evaluate the meaning of sensations and affective states, discriminate present from past, and to interpret social cues in the context of current realities rather than the past events.

Traumas and people can be so uniquely different and the ability to compare information may not necessarily be generalizable. It appears that a dependable method of research is the Self-Report Data of the victims, but that can also be fraught with bias.

Another difficulty is the appropriate selection to mirror the extreme or unique traumatic event. Such groups present a threat to the validity of the research design. For instance, divorce has become more common, so studies on divorce and the inherent trauma are becoming more common.

> Without the option of inflicting actual trauma in the laboratory, there are only limited options for the exploration of traumatic memories, by collecting retrospective reports from traumatized individuals, post hoc observations or provoking of a traumatic memory and flashback in people with PTSD. (Fisler, 1995).

The personal narrative of patients, which involves explicit memory, is sometimes of questionable validity in the understanding of trauma.

Chapter 3

<u>Methodology</u>

<u>Introduction</u>

This study focuses on trauma, which refers to;

> "…the state of a person being violated, often by someone on whom they depended and having their trust broken, feeling helpless, vulnerable, disabled or threatened with death" (Yehuda, et al., 1997).

The professional and familial caregivers effects following a minimum of four years after the event will be explored. It is clear that there are other people and situations that are not addressed by this research, but for the sake of this study, these parameters provide boundaries for the research design. The quantitative tests serve to establish the finding of secondary traumatization for caregivers of trauma. These results will work in conjunction with the qualitative instruments to describe the participants experiences and perceptions as they relate to Post Traumatic Stress Disorder and Resiliency factors.

The study used a battery of two quantitative self-report tests with high reliability and validity and two open-ended qualitative tests to discover key factors in resiliency among caregivers with secondary traumatization in a one-contact cross-sectional design. This study has examined protective factors and resiliency factors. Borg and Gall propose a "...strategy of using several different kinds of data-collection instruments, such as tests, direct observations, interviews, and content analysis, to explore a single problem or issue" (1989, p. 393).

The participants were self-selected volunteers responding to posters in area hospitals as well as collegial referrals. The surveys were administered to 20 familial caretakers, 20 professional caretakers, and 20 people in a control group.

Van Der Kolk's Trauma Studies Institute in Boston has developed a trauma assessment package that consistings of two different instruments. This study employed the pencil test called the Modified PTSD Symptoms Scale (Van Der Kolk, 1994). The purpose of the test is to assist the clinician to ascertain if the participant has PTSD. The test will evaluate the level of symptomotology in the patient and help to also organize a treatment plan that is specific to the patient's needs. The approach in the present study is to measure instead the level of emotional stress on the caregivers and the resiliency factors that allow them to continue in the caregiving battle.

The quantitative hypotheses for this study are;

(1) There will be significant differences on PTSD scores in familial and professional caregivers compared to control participants consistent with secondary traumatization.

(2) "There is an inverse relationship, between the two measures of resiliency and PTSD.

(3) There will be gender effects on familial and professional caregivers PTSD scores.

Van Der Kolk and the Trauma Center designed the PTSD Symptom Scale that "...specifically inquires about the sensory, affective and narrative voice of remembering the triggers for unbidden recollections of traumatic memories, and ways of mastering unwanted intrusions of traumatic memories. (Van Der Kolk & Fisler, 1995). This 17 item scale structures the interview and collects data about the circumstances around a person's trauma, its nature, what led to it, what senses they were feeling at that time, whether they have nightmares, a confirmation through documentation of records, and other data. The PTSD Symptom Scale takes half an hour to administer and is then analyzed to compare data. There are two sub-samples of groups, the 60 participants for the qualitative tests and the eight participants for the qualitative in-depth interviews.

Research Design

Data Collection

The method used for this study involved a post-treatment assessment/test with a control group. Assessments were made following the actual caregiving experience. The data collection process made use of 2 objective quantitative tests and one open-ended qualitative in-depth interview of 8 caretakers (4 professional and 4 familial). Also, the 20 professional and 20 familial caretakers answered 6 brief narrative questions (see Appendix A) as part of the researcher's efforts to better understand the experience and emotional impact of caregiving and resiliency. This one-time assessment and study used 2 quantitative scales and 2 qualitative in-depth interviews. The quantitative PTSD symptom multiple choice questionnaire and the resilience/hardiness scale have high validity and reliability as noted on p. 78. The third instrument was a qualitative semi-structured in-depth interview for a smaller number of participants (n=8) that addresses the participants' ability to cope with the daily stressors of professional caregiving. The protocol followed Kvale (1996) for guidance on qualitative interviews. These interviews were tape-recorded and used all the questions from the resiliency questionnaire (see Appendix B). The qualitative results will establish if the participants have PTSD and they will inform the quantitative result by describing in the participants personal experience and recommendations for other caregivers.

The research questions for qualitative in-depth interviews were:

(1) Does the caretaking experience include features of secondary traumatization and what are the major difficulties of this experience?

(2) What is the nature of risk factors that aggravate and protective factors that eliminate the difficulties of the caretaking experience?

(3) What part do spirituality and hope play in resiliency for caregivers?

(4) What do professional and familial caregivers recommend to others to help them sustain the caregiving battle?

These questions are designed to elicit information to determine whether the caregiver is suffering symptoms of secondary traumatization, the impact of gender issues, social connectedness, self-esteem, and spirituality. The qualitative interview was designed to study the subjective expectations and psychological outcomes of caregiving for a person with traumatic or chronic illness. Miles and Huberman (1994) state,

> Initial choices of informants lead you to similar and different ones; observing one class of events invites comparison with another; and understanding one key relationship within the setting reveals facets to be studied in others. This is a conceptually-driven sequential sampling. (p.27)

This study required a sample population of caregivers that are the articulate and interested in resiliency factors of the caregiving role so that we may compare commonalities of responses. The first round of interviews presented a series of 8 open-ended questions to the 8 participants. These questions provided a narrative of information about this deeply human experience and what caregiving has meant to them.

Participants

The participants for both the quantitative survey portion and the in-depth segment, were voluntary and were recruited from level-one trauma centers in Boston, and New York. The recruiting mechanism for both substudies was a letter, posted in the family waiting areas and staff lounges, that requested volunteers for a study of key factors in resiliency for subjects in extended caregiving capacities (see Appendix C). Other letters were placed in rehabilitation center support groups in the metropolitan area and some participants were recruited through collegial recommendations that they volunteer. Each participant completed a consent form (see Appendix D).

The 60 study participants included 20 familial and 20 professional caregivers, plus 20 members of a control group. Each participant responded voluntarily and were obtained by self-selection. The participants for the in-depth interviews consisted of the first eight that responded or voluntered. Both men and women were included as participants in this study, but they were not stratified. The research design required that the participants (except in the control group) had been in the role of caregiver in a familial or professional capacity for a minimum of four years following a traumatic episode. The study selected specifically for people who were experienced in the pitfalls and rewards of caregiving for a patient. The participants had progressed through the initial grieving and shock period and stabilized to a daily routine. The participants were required to be willing and able to disclose their feelings, both negative and positive, to the researcher. The participants were advised that the interview process might contribute to their emotional distress and were advised that referrals would be given to anyone who appeared to be depressed or in need of clinical treatment for independent evaluation and follow-up.

This study attempted to understand the resiliency traits in caregivers as a general group. This random study approach made use of "People who are uniquely able to be informative because they are expert in an area or were privileged witnesses to an event" (Weiss, 1994, p.17.)

Instruments

The quantitative portion of the study consisted of a battery of two self-report questionnaires and psychological tests. The first test by Van Der Kolk is the Modified PTSD Symptom Scale, which is a 17-item questionnaire that asks respondents the frequency and intensity of their symptoms. This instrument was used for the DSM-IV trials on Post Traumatic Stress Disorder (Van Der Kolk, 1995). The content validity questions, address how trauma exposure manifested in PTSD symptoms for the patient. This test consists of questions regarding the participants' past and current functioning, such as affect regulation, re-experiencing, dissociation, and hyper-vigilance.

The study also used the Dispositional Resiliency Scale (DRS) by Bartone and Ursano (1989), which measures the emotional context of the participant's with regard to illness, anxiety, depression, and coping mechanisms. The DRS consists of 45 items on a Likert-type scale and is intended to measure resiliency based on the participants' commitment, spirituality/hope, and self-esteem of the participant. The Bartone and Ursano study was conducted in 1985 and was designed to measure the impact of the health of workers following an airline disaster in Newfoundland. It also measures personality style and the power of endurance as factors in resilience.

The final qualitative measure for 8 participants was an in-depth interview that elicited the participant's feelings, perceptions, and coping skills relative to their caregiving duties. The questions were based on the findings of the literature review; the interviews were tape-recorded. In addition, the 20 familial and professional caregivers responded to 6 written qualitative brief questions (see Appendix A). The caregivers perceptions and recommendations for other caregivers were explored. The study hoped to reveal protective/risk factors that would allow the caretakers to sustain the caregiving experience such as social supports, spirituality and self-esteem.

<u>Procedures</u>

The participants met with the researcher for one half hour prior to being given the test. The research setting was the general hospital's psychiatry clinic in which observations were made. Participants received a packet that contained the one qualitative and two quantitative tests and the informed consent to participate form. They had one week to complete the tests and return them in a self-addressed stamped envelope that was included in the packet. The semi-structured interviews were done at the hospital with 8 voluntary participants. The interviews were tape-recorded and drew on the questions shown in Appendix A.

The researcher offered to meet with each participant two weeks after the initial interview to answer questions and receive feedback.

<u>Data Analysis</u>

The data analysis for both sub-studies was conducted following the completion of the interviews. The study examined descriptive statistics by subgroup.

Two quantitative self-report questionnaires; the PTSD Symptom Scale, the Resiliency/Hardiness Scale provided data consisting of the scores of the two variables, means, and standard deviations. They were analyzed to assess for coping efficiency and resiliency. The analysis procedure for the quantitative tests involved coding and scoring according to a score sheet provided by the authors of the two tests. These quantitative tests compared data regarding primary symptoms to those of secondary traumatization symptoms presented by professional and familial caregivers.

The qualitative written questions for the 60 participant's and in-depth interviews for the 8 participant's were explored for commonalities and issues significant to the participants' resiliency. The researcher studied the participant's attitudes, emotions, and behavioral changes of the participants as self-reported for the entire caregiving process or period. The variables considered were endurance, adaptation, resiliency, self-esteem, social connectedness, hardiness, role models, professional emotional distance, insight, and ability to articulate feelings.

The analysis of the qualitative data was studied to identify patterns and common themes in the data. This exploratory theory approach was used to test a hypothesis of resiliency factors among caregivers and to obtain a conceptual and personal understanding of the participants' experience and lived meanings. The approach examines the participants' attitudes, emotions, and behavioral changes throughout the process of caregiving.

The methodology of quantitative and qualitative self-report measures assessed the psychological impact of secondary traumatization and sequelae. The posttraumatic data adaptation evaluations were analyzed using SAS 8.2 that assists the researcher in the statistical analysis of the data. The figures and graphs will be constructed with the assistance of Microsoft Excel. These quantitative and qualitative tests combined to inform the research about possible secondary traumatization of the participants and the key factors in their power of endurance, adaptability, and resiliency.

Chapter 4

Results

<u>Quantitative Analysis</u>

The dependent variable for this study is the level of PTSD from the quantitative Modified PTSD Symptom Scale and the independent variables are gender, caretaker groups and resiliency as assessed by the Resiliency/Hardiness Scale. The participant population (N = 60) consisted of 20 familial caregivers, 20 members of a control group, and 20 professional caregivers. This chapter presents separate analyses of the variables for control group, professional caregivers, and family caregiver, individually and compared with each other. The findings represent the results of the data from all participants. When the tests for the PTSD Symptom Scale and the resiliency scale were scored, the researcher tested the hypothesis that caregivers of trauma victims exhibited higher PTSD scores. Three sets of t-tests were conducted to compare the means of variable PTSD score for each pair of caregiver groups. Then three 3x2 analyses of variance (ANOVA) and Scheffe's contrast tests were performed to test whether caregiving or resiliency affect the tendency of developing PTSD symptoms. Pearson Correlation was also carried out to determine the degree to which resiliency was associated with the tendency of getting PTSD symptoms. The study also used Pearson Correlation to determine the degree to which the dependent variables of resiliency were associated, as well as an analysis of variance (ANOVA) to determine the impact of gender as a dependent variable on the results. Tables and graphs throughout this chapter will present the appropriate means, standard deviations, degrees of freedom, and significance for each of the variables tested.

I. Preliminary analyses

Table 1 below provides the demographic breakdown for the study participants.

Demographics of Quantitative Study Participants

Gender		Ethnicity		Therapy	Education		Income	
Control Group								
Female	11	Cauc	14	Yes 2	HS 11		15-25K	8
55%		70%		10%	55%		25-50K	3
		Asian	4		College 4		50-100K	6
Male	9	20%		No 18	20%		100-500K	3
45%		Afro-Amer 1		90%	Ms 5			
		5%			25%			
		Amer-Ind 1			Other 1			
		5%			5%			
Family Caregivers								
Female	6	Cauc	19	Yes 11	HS 6		15-25K	1
30%		95%		55%	30%		25-50K	5
					College 7		50-100K	5
Male	14	Afric-Amer 1		No 9	35%		100-500K	5
70%		5%		45%	MD 1		At home	4
					5%			
					MS 5			
					25%			
					PHD 1			
					5%			
Professional Caregivers								
Female	10	Cauc	18	Yes 19	HS	2	15-25K	3
50%		90%		95%	10%		25-50K	1
		Asian	2	No 1	College 4		50-100K	4
Male	10	10%		5%	20%		100-500 K	12
50%					PhD	2		
					10%			
					MD	12		
					60%			

N=60

II. Hypothesis Testing

The following examines the distribution of PTSD scores to test the quantitative hypothesis.

Hypothesis 1

"There will be significant differences on PTSD scores in familial and professional caregivers compared to control participants consistent with secondary traumatization."

The Modified PTSD Symptom Scale test results revealed that PTSD symptoms are more prevalent in familial and professional caregivers than in the control population according group comparisons. However, before doing the comparisons, the distribution of the data needed to be determined. If there is a normal distribution, a t test or chi-square test can be used in the comparison.

Table 2

Mean Scores for Variable PTSD

Group	N	M	SD
Control	20	7.10	7.10
Familial	20	24.15	26.69
Prof.	20	18.05	9.18

Note. N=60

Figure 1a gives the mean of the PTSD scores for each group. The mean values for familial and professional caregivers are higher than those of the controls. Figure 1b shows the box plots of the PTSD score distribution. First quartile (25th percentile) and third quartile (75th percentile) are shown by lower and upper edge of box, respectively. Median (50th percentile) is represented by the line inside box. Mean is shown by the blue symbol marker.

Figure 1.   **PTSD Scores By Group**

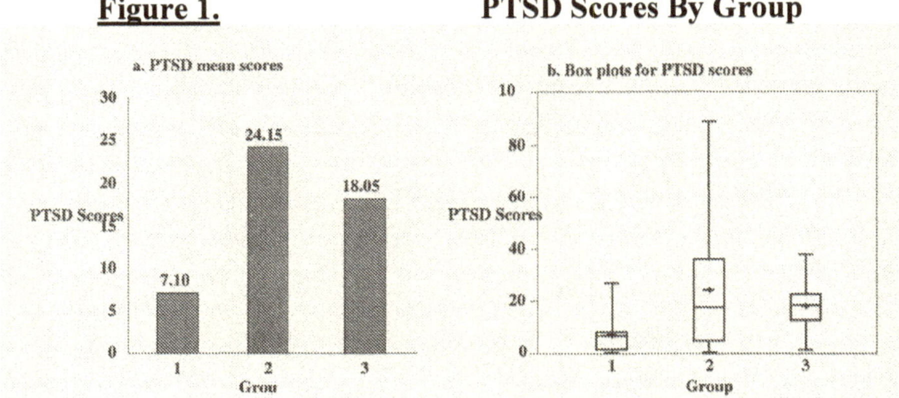

Figure 1. Mean scores for PTSD Symptoms by Group 1: Controls; Group 2: Familial caregivers; Group 3: Professional caregivers. N=60

Figure 1a represents the resiliency mean scores for each group. Figure 1b represents the maximum resiliency score and the minimum resiliency score as demonstrated by the box plots for each group.

Table 3

Means for Variable PTSD and Resiliency Classified by Variable
Group and Gender

Level of Gender	Level of Group	PTSD			Resiliency		
		N	M	SD	N	M	SD
Male	Controls	11	6.55	7.06	11	52.18	9.26
Male	Familial	6	21.17	18.77	6	44.00	14.37
Male	Prof	11	13.91	7.25	11	50.64	12.92
Female	Controls	9	7.78	7.51	9	49.44	8.03
Female	Familial	14	25.43	30.00	14	49.50	9.20
Female	Prof	9	23.11	9.06	9	48.11	7.59

Note. N=60

The Modified PTSD Symptom Scale test results revealed that

PTSD symptoms are more prevalent in familial and professional

caregivers than in the normal population according t test group

comparisons. Before the t-tests, testing equality of variances for the

Susan Cooney, Ph.D.

paired groups is necessary. Only the variances of controls and

professional caregivers are equal (Table 3).

Table 3.1   Equality of Variances for Variable PTSD

Group	df	F	P
Controls vs. Familial caregivers	19	14.13	<.0001
Controls vs. Professional caregivers	19	1.67	0.27
Familial vs. Professional caregivers	19	8.46	<.0001

Note. N=60

Table 4   t-Test for PTSD Score by Group

Caregiver Group	N	M	SD	df	t	P
Control vs. Familial Group	20	7.10	1.55	38	-2.76***	0.01*
Control vs. Professional Group	20	24.15	3.33	38	-4.22***	0.00***
Familial vs. Professional Group	20	18.05	1.55	38	.97	0.34

Note. N=60 *p<.05. **p<.01. ***p<.001

Table 4 shows the t-test results.

The hypotheses for two-sided tests are:

1. Controls & Familial caregivers:

H_0: Controls and Familial caregivers have the same tendency for PTSD

H$_a$: They have different tendencies for PTSD

    2. Controls & Professional caregivers:

H$_0$: Controls and Professional caregivers have the same tendency for PTSD

H$_a$: They have different tendencies for PTSD

    3. Familial caregivers & Professional caregivers:

H$_0$: Familial caregivers and Professional caregivers have the same tendency for PTSD

H$_a$: They have different tendencies for PTSD

The methods used and the corresponding results are shown in bold. The *p* value for controls and familiar caregivers, 0.01, is less than 0.05, which results in rejection of the null hypothesis. Contrasting PTSD scores for controls vs. familial caregivers yeilded $t(38)=-2.76$, $p<.01$. Thus, familial caregivers are more prone to get PTSD compared to people without frequent contact with PTSD patients. The same holds true for professional caregivers yeilded $t(38)=-4.22$, $p<.01$. Thus, hypothesis 1 is true; "Professional and familial caregivers will show significantly higher PTSD scores than the control participants." Meanwhile, we compared the PTSD scores of familial and professional caregivers. $P<0.34$, much larger than

0.05, which indicates that the tendency to get PTSD is not significantly different between familial or professional caregivers.

Scheffe's Test for PTSD on Group

Table 5.1 Mean Difference at Significance level of 0.05

Comparison	Difference Between Means	Simultaneous 95% Confidence Limits		Minimum Significant Difference of Mean
Caregiver F, Caregivers P	6.10	- 7.42*	19.62	13.52
Caregivers F, Controls P	17.05	3.52	30.57	13.52
Caregivers F, Controls P	10.95	- 2.57*	24.47	13.52

Note: Comparisons significant at the *p< 0.05 level. N=60

5.2 Scheffe Grouping on Caregivers

Scheffe Grouping	M	N	GROUP
A	24.15	20	Familial
B	18.05	20	Professional
B	7.10	20	Controls

Note: Means with the same letter are not significantly different. N=60

Table =0.05 by□5.1 presents the mean difference and the minimum mean difference at Scheffe's test. In table 5.2, means with the same letter are not significantly different. It seems that gender has no effect on PTSD symptoms (Table 5.2), and familial caregivers have significantly higher PTSD than the normal population (Table 5.2). Female professional caregivers had a significantly greater tendency to get PTSD, their mean PTSD scores was higher than that of the normal population (Table 5.1).

A 3x2 ANOVA was conducted, taking PTSD scores as dependent variable (DV), caregiver group, gender and their interaction as the independent variables (IV) (Table 9). Whether the other effects were adjusted, it shows that the p value for group effect is less than 0.05, confirming hypothesis 1 holds true. On the other hand, the p values for gender, or gender and group interaction are larger than 0.05, suggesting that both male and female have the same tendency of developing PTSD symptoms. However, it appears that gender has some effect on PTSD scores in professional caregivers (p value = 0.02

< 0.05, but not in controls (*p* value = 0.71; see or familial caregivers

(*p* value = 0.75) table 6.2.

Table 6.1

3 X 2 ANOVA Table for PTSD Scores by Group and Gender

Level of Gender	Caretaker Group	PTSD Scores		
		N	M	SD
Male	Controls	11	6.55	7.06
Male	Familial caregivers	6	21.17	18.77
Male	Prof caregivers	11	13.91	7.25
Female	Controls	9	7.78	7.51
Female	Familial caregivers	14	25.43	30.00
Female	Prof caregivers	9	23.11	9.06

Note: N= 60

ANOVA Table for PTSD Scores by Group and Gender

6.2 Main Effect and Interaction

Source	N	df	SS	MS	F	P
Gender	6	1	783.00	783.00	2.71	0.10

	0					
Group	6 0	2	2545.5 0	1272.75	4.41	0.01*
Gender*Gro up	6 0	2	159.89	79.95	0.28	0.75

Note. N=60   *p<.05. **p<.01. ***p<.001

Hypothesis 2

"There is an inverse relationship, between the two measures of resiliency and PTSD."

Multiple tests were conducted for variable Resiliency scores. Thus, the T test results are shown in (Table 7). The results show that *p* values for control group vs. professional groups is much larger than 0.05, indicating that resiliency is not very different amongst the two groups. However, the familial group compared with professional and control groups, has significantly less resiliency.

Table 7.1

Equality of Variances for Variable Resiliency

Caregiver Group	df	F	P

Controls vs. Familial caregivers	19	1.60	0.31
Controls vs. Professional caregivers	19	1.53	0.35
Familial vs. Professional caregivers	19	1.05	0.92

Note. N=60 *p<.05

Table 7.2

<u>t-Test for Resiliency Scores by Group</u>

Caregiver Group	N	M	SD	df	t	P
Control vs. Familial Group	20	50.95	8.62	38	1.00	0.32
Control vs. Professional Group	20	47.85	10.91	38	0.47	0.63
Familial vs. Professional Group	20	49.50	10.67	38	- 0.48	0.63

Note. N=60 *p<.05. **p<.01. ***p<.001

Similarly, a 3x2 ANOVA was done for Resiliency as DV, caregiver group, gender and their interaction as IV's (Table 8). The *p* values for group interaction is less than 0.05, confirming the results from t-test that resiliency was not different among control and professional caregiver groups, but a slightly less for familial caregivers. It also indicates no gender effect on resiliency. The results showed a significant difference in resiliency among familial caregivers as compared to professional and control groups. The dependent variable is resiliency, with two levels of gender (male and female), and three levels of caretaker group (control, Familial, Professional caretakers) as independent variables.

ANOVA Table for Resiliency by Group and Gender

8.1 Whole Model Effect

Source	df	SS	MS	F	P
Model	5	291.94	58.39	0.56	0.730
Error	54	5638.80	104.42		
Corrected Total	59	5930.73			

Note. N=60 *p<.05. **p<.01. ***p<.001

ANOVA Table for Resiliency by Group and Gender
8.2 Main Effects and Interaction

Source	N	df	SS	MS	F	P
Gender	60	1	7.91	7.91	0.08	0.78
Caregiver/Control	60	2	88.94	44.47	0.43	0.65
Gender*Group	60	2	195.09	97.54	0.93	0.39

Note. N=60 *p<.05. **p<.01. ***p<.001

For analysis of Resiliency, there was a nonsignificant main effect

on gender with F(1,54)=0.08 (p<.78) and a nonspecific main effect on

Caregiver group with F(2,54)= 0.43, and a nonsignificant interaction

F(2,54)=0.93 for gender/group.

Table 9   <u>Means and Standard Deviations For Variable PTSD</u>

<u>Classified by Group and Resiliency n=60</u>

Resiliency	Group	PTSD		
		N	Mean	Std Dev
Low	Controls	8	7.37	4.65
Low	Familial	10	14.00	16.73
Low	Professional	12	21.16	9.41
High	Controls	12	6.91	8.55
High	Familial	10	34.30	31.54

| High | Professional | 8 | 13.37 | 6.90 |

To test the relationship of PTSD symptoms with coping strength (resiliency) or gender, the study used ANOVA. The null hypothesis states that there is an association between resiliency and PTSD scores, as well as between gender and PTSD scores. The researcher further used the Pearson correlation test to confirm the results of the ANOVA and detail the relationship between resiliency and PTSD scores, and between gender and PTSD scores.

Also, as demonstrated by Table 12, there is a negative correlation between resiliency and PTSD scores. However, it appears that gender has some effect on PTSD scores in professional caregivers (p value = 0.02 < 0.05), but not in controls (p value = 0.71); see or familial caregivers (p value = 0.75).

Table 10

<u>ANOVA Table for PTSD Scores on Group and Resiliency</u>

10.1 Whole Model Effect

Source	df	SS	MS	**F**	**P**
Model	5	5338.30	1067.66	4.20	0.002*

			**
Error	54	13742.43	254.48
Corrected Total	59	19080.73	

Note: n=60 *p<.05. **p<.01. ***p<.001

10.2 Main Effect and Interaction

Source	df	SS	MS	F	P
Resiliency	1	106.67	106.67	0.42	0.52
Caregiver/Control Group	2	3141.21	1570.60	6.17	0.003***
Resiliency*Group	2	2090.43	1045.21	4.11	0.02*

Note: n=60 *p<.05. **p<.01. ***p<.001

We examined the relation between resiliency and PTSD scores by a 3x2 ANOVA taking PTSD scores, with three levels of group (control, professional and familial caretaker) and two levels of resiliency and PTSD symptoms. The result is shown in table 10. Resiliency was categorized as lower (less or equal to the mean) and higher (greater than the mean) levels. The group effect exists according to both the ANOVA (*p* value is 0.006 after adjustment of other effects, table 10.2). However, *p* value for resiliency is 0.34 after adjustment of other effects (table 10.2), indicating that higher resiliency does not lower the development of PTSD symptoms. Although the *p* value for interaction between resiliency and group is less than 0.05, it means only the group difference affects PTSD symptom development.

Table 11 <u>Scheffe's Test for Resiliency on Group</u>

Mean Difference at Significance level of 0.05

Comparison	Difference Between Means	Simultaneous 95% Confidence Limits		Minimum Significant Difference of Mean
Caregivers (F) Caregivers (P)	-1.65*	-9.78	6.84	8.13
Caregivers(F) Controls	-3.10*	-11.23	5.03	8.13
Caregivers(P) Controls	-1.45*	-9.58	6.68	8.13

Note: Comparisons significant at the *p<0.05 level. N=60

Pearson Correlation test was later conducted to further explore if higher resiliency affected PTSD scores. Resiliency had *p* values > 0.05, which suggests no rejection of the null hypothesis that resiliency had no effect on PTSD scores of familial caregivers comparing to controls (Table 12). Further, resiliency appears to have some correlation with PTSD scores in professional caregivers with a P value = 0.06). The Pearson correlation coefficient is -0.35 (Table

12b), which indicates that the more resilient a professional caregiver is, the less chance of developing PTSD, as would be normally expected.

Table 12

Pearson Correlation of Resiliency and PTSD Scores

12a) Test of H_0: Pearson Correlation = 0

	Group		
	Controls	Familial caregivers	Professional caregivers
pr	0.3865	0.2038	0.06

Note. N=60 *p<.05. **p<.01. ***p<.001

12.b Pearson Correlation Coefficient of Resiliency and PTSD Scores by Caretaker Group

	Caregiver Groups		
	Controls	Familial caregivers	Professional caregivers
Correlation(r)	-0.06	0.15	-0.35 **
95% Lower CI	-0.47	-0.20	-0.79**
95% Upper CI	0.35	0.51	0.09*

Note. N=60 *p<.05. **p<.01. ***p<.001

High resiliency seems to have no effect on PTSD scores in controls or familial caregivers, with *p* values > 0.05. Further, resiliency appears to have some relationship with PTSD scores in professional caregivers p<.10 level (*p* value= 0.06). The Pearson correlation coefficient is -0.35, which indicates that the higher the resiliency a professional caregiver has, the less chance he has of getting PTSD, as would be normally expected. There could possibly be a higher significance if the study had a higher n. Surprisingly, this study discovered a negative correlation between resiliency and PTSD scores.

Hypothesis 3

"There will be a gender effects on familial and professional caregivers PTSD scores."

Gender mean, values, and distribution are shown in Figure 3. The familial caregiver group had more males than females; however, the difference had minimal impact on the reliability of the following tests for the gender effect. The rank procedure was performed before the

ANOVA test for gender.

Figure 3 demonstrates the combined total scores for the Modified

PTSD Symptom Scale and the Resliency Scale by Group and gender.

The highest score is 74.93 for the female familial caretaker.

Figure 3: Histogram of Combined PTSD and Resiliency Scores by Gender and Group

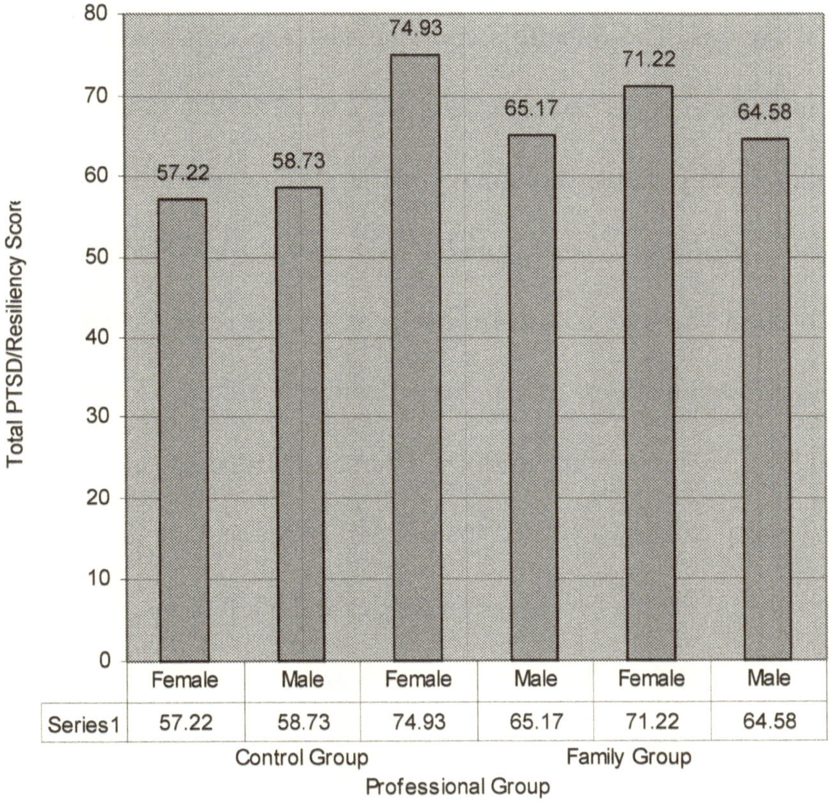

	Female	Male	Female	Male	Female	Male
Series1	57.22	58.73	74.93	65.17	71.22	64.58

Control Group Professional Group Family Group

Note. N-60

To test the relationship of PTSD symptoms with resiliency and gender, the study conducted an ANOVA. The familial caregiver group had more males than females; however, the difference was not significant enough to impact on the reliability of ANOVA for the gender effect. The null hypothesis states that there is an association between resiliency and PTSD scores, as well as between gender and PTSD scores. The Scheffe's contrasts test was conducted to test the mean difference of the six cells of 3x2 ANOVA. The researcher further performed the Pearson correlation test to detail the relationship between resiliency, gender and PTSD scores. A typical goal in an analysis of variance is to compare means of the response variable for various combinations of the classification variables. Following the ANOVA, the researcher used the Pearson correlation test to confirm the results of the ANOVA for gender effect and to determine the nature of the correlation between gender and PTSD scores.

The model for ANOVA is PTSD scores $= b_0 + \text{Gender} * b_1$ and the null hypothesis is $b_1 = 0$.

The null hypothesis states that there will be no significant main effects or interactions of Resiliency, as a function of gender or Caretaker Group.

ANOVA Table for Resiliency by Group and Gender

8.2 Main Effect and Interaction

Source	N	df	SS	MS	F	P
Gender	60	1	7.91	7.91	0.08	0.78
Caregiver/Control Group	60	2	88.94	44.47	0.43	0.65
Gender*Group	60	2	195.09	97.54	0.93	0.39

Note n=60 *p<.05. **p<.01. ***p<.001

Table 13 <u>Scheffe's Test for PTSD on Gender</u>

13a Mean Difference at Significance level of 0.05

Gender Comparison	Difference Between Means	Simultaneous 95% Confidence Limits		Minimum Significant Difference of Mean
Female – Male	7.24	- 1.57	16.05	8.81

N=60

13b Scheffe Grouping on Gender

Scheffe Grouping	M	N	Gender
Equal Variances Assumed	19.81	32	Female
	12.57	28	Male

Note: N=60

Scheffe's Test for Resiliency on Gender

14.2a Mean Difference at Significance level of 0.05

Gender Comparison	Difference Between Means	Simultaneous 95% Confidence Limits	Minimum Significant Difference of Mean
Female – Male	-0.77	- 4.57 6.02	5.30

Note: N=60

Following the ANOVA and Scheffe gender tests, the researcher performed the Pearson correlation test to check the correlation between gender and resiliency and PTSD scores.

Table 12 Pearson Correlation of Resiliency and PTSD Scores by gender

12a) Test of H_0: Pearson Correlation = 0

	Gender	
	male	Female
pr	0.1186	0.4627

Note N=60 *$p<.05$. **$p<.01$. ***$p<.001$

FIGURE 1C: MODIFIED PTSD SYMPTOM SCALE

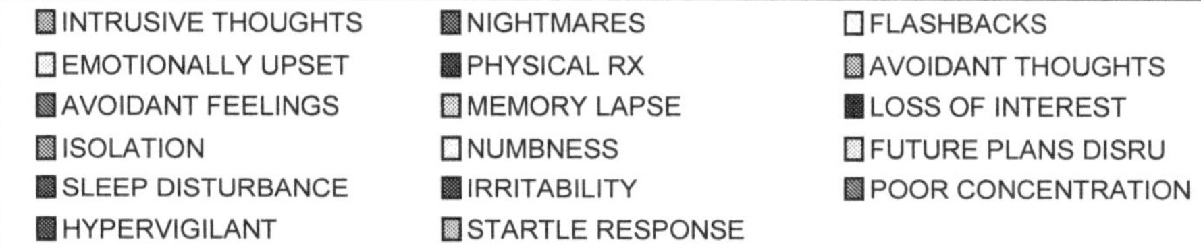

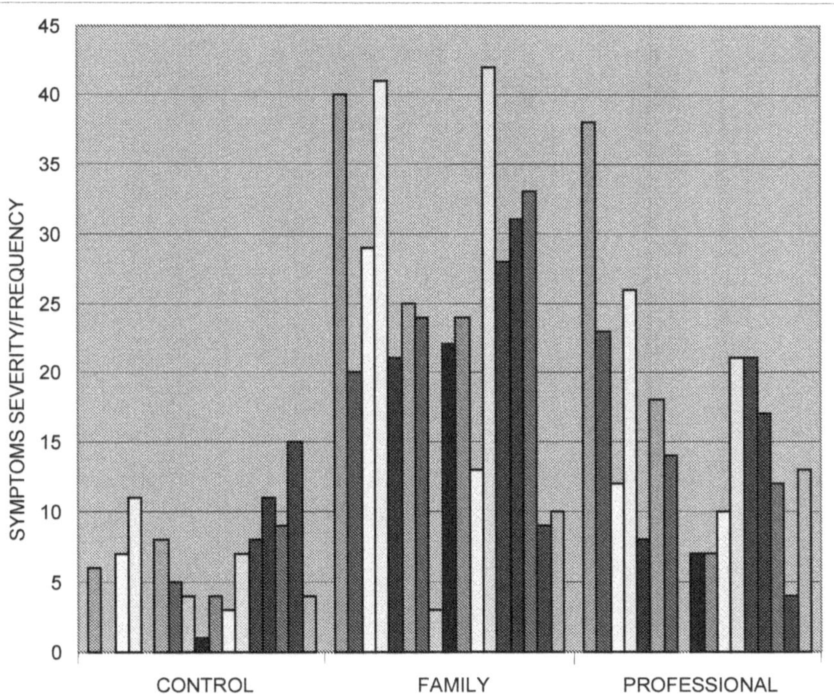

FIGURE 2C: RESILIENCY SCALE SCORES
PIE CHART BY GROUP

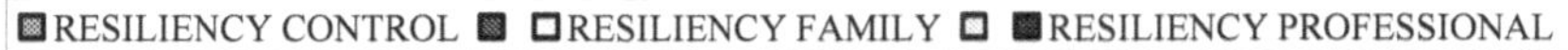

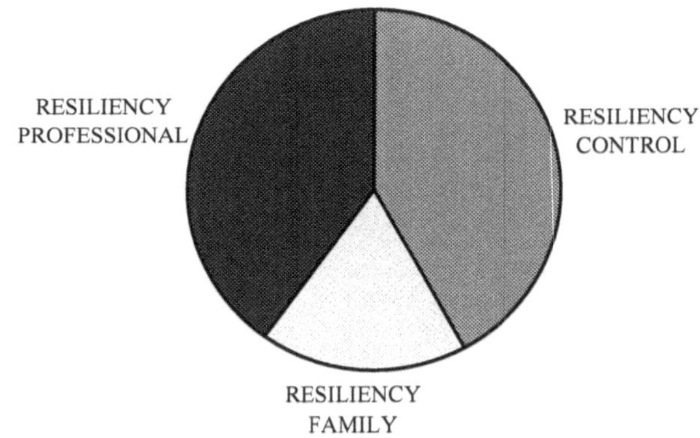

Note. N=60 Total Resiliency Scale scores by control and Professional and Familial caretaker groups.

FIGURE 2

Resiliency Scores by Group

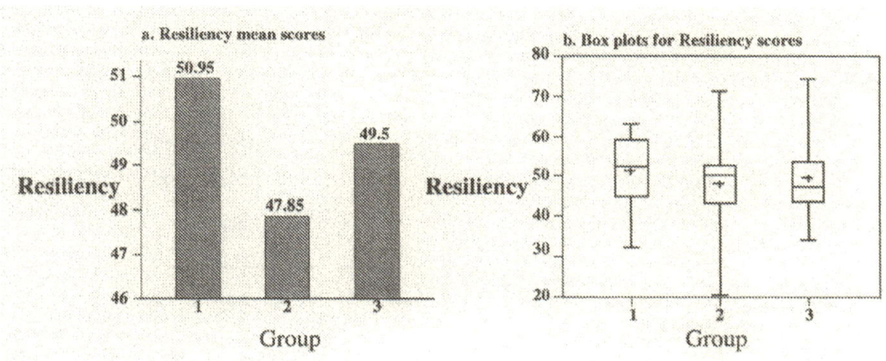

Figure 2 : Mean resiliency scores by Group 1: Controls; Group 2: Familial caregivers; Group 3: Professional caregivers.

N=60

Figure 2a represents the resiliency mean scores for each group.

Figure 2b represents the maximum resiliency score and the minimum

resiliency score as demonstrated by the box plots for each group.

Results of the Qualitative Semi-structured Interviews

<u>Demographics of Qualitative Interview Study Participants</u>

Table 1.1

Gender	Ethnicity	Therapy	Education	Income
Professional Group				
Female 1 25%	Cauc 4 100%	Yes 2 50%	HS College	15-25K 25-50K
	Asian	No 2 50%	Ms 1 25%	50-100K 1
Male 3 75%	Afro-Amer		MD 3 75%	100-500K 3
	Amer-Ind		PhD	
Family Caregivers				
Female 3 75%	Cauc 4 100%	Yes 1 25%	HS College 4 100%	15-25K 25-50K 1 50-100K 2
	Asian			
Male 1 25%	Afric-Amer	No 3 75%	MD	100-500K 1
	Ameri-Ind		MS	At home
			PhD	

N=8

<u>Overview of the Interviewees</u>

The qualitative results are based on interviews with 8 caregivers, 4 of whom were familial and 4 professional caregivers. There were 4 male and 4 female participants, who varied in age from 28 to 67. The participants were voluntary and the first eight who responded for the interview were accepted. Unfortunately, there isn't any ethnic diversity for the in-depth interview section of the study. The results of the semi-structured qualitative question, are based on the participants' knowledge in response to each question (Appendix A). Quotations are be included on occasion to capture the essence of their experience. They gave permission to include their narrative vignettes as long as their identities were not revealed.

Interviewee 1 is a 41-year-old married male and a family caregiver to his mother, who has suffered from illness for 25 years and is often in critical condition. He states he felt duty bound to care for her because of love and necessity. This has, however, affected his social interactions, and he feels that he is developmentally delayed. His drive to "do the right thing" propels him on.

Interviewee 2 is a 43-year-old female family caregiver. She has recently lost the family member for whom she was caring and is tearful and grieving. She says that the process of caregiving was exhausting, but makes it clear that she would never have stopped had the patient lived. She reports focusing on resources and research to find medical options as a coping mechanism. She feels that "hope is the catalyst that keeps you going."

Interviewee 3 is a 47-year-old married physician and family caregiver to a mother and brother. He feels that balancing his life with exercise and friends and his spirituality have been a driving force. He speculates that because he is in the medical field that he may be able to distance himself from the emotional component a little more successfully. He admits, however, that there were times with his mother's and brother's illnesses that he was overwhelmed.

Interviewee 4 is a 44-year-old married female family caregiver. She cared for her brother until his death at the age of 30. She is mystical and spiritual in her outlook. She was fiercely determined to make her brother comfortable and to explore all medical options. She says that she could not allow her emotions to rule even though she wanted to fall apart and that she needed to focus on what needed to be done and help her parents through the ordeal. It took a toll on her emotionally and physically, and she says, "You go on, but you never get over it."

Interviewee 5 is a 69-year-old married male trauma surgeon. His work has exposed him to some of the most difficult and sad scenarios. He is philosophical and able to find a balance between caring and being able to perform his job. He says, "It breaks your heart sometimes, but you have to find a way to balance so that you can take care of the patients." When asked what he recommends to new trainees for coping, he stoically reports, "Everyone has to find their own way. However, every time you have a win, it helps you deal with the losses. So, I tell them to just keep working, that is all you can do."

Interviewee 6 is a 33-year-old single female nurse who is also a familial caregiver. She was reserved, guarded, and anxious. She was tearful throughout the qualitative in-depth interview. At the end of the interview, however, she reported feeling better for having talked about it. She cared for her dying mother for many years all by herself. Her sister lived in another state and her father had passed away. She reported that the hours were long and the treatments were overwhelming but she kept going, "...because I had to and because I wanted to."

Interviewee 7 is a 40-year-old married male trauma surgeon. He seems a bit impatient and gruff. He said that his confidence in his skill and the rewards of helping people sustained him. He scoffs at the idea that he becomes emotionally involved with his patients and their lives.

Yet, he scored significantly high on the PTSD symptom scale. He stated that, " it becomes easier to emotionally distance yourself as the years go by. He accepts that as long as you do your clinical best for your patient, no matter how it turns out, then you must move on to the next patient, that there are no other options and you have to keep going because someone else needs your help."

Interviewee 8 is a 37-year-old married female familial caregiver to a 9-year-old son who was in a near-drowning accident. He has been in a persistent vegetative state since he was four. She admits to isolation as a result of her son's needs. She appears to draw strength from her interactions with her son; although he is unresponsive, she feels he understands. She said that she is surprised by her knowledge and medical competency surrounding his condition and requirements. She is able to suction him, change dressings, and monitor his vital signs. She feels that her faith and hope keep her going. She says that her faith buffers her against despair, and she trusts there is a reason for what has happened.

Qualitative Semi-Structured Interview Analysis

This section presents the analyses of the qualitative semi-structured interviews with familial and professional caregivers.

Interview Question 1. What inspired or led you to become a caregiver?

The research design allowed respondents to this questionnaire to answer in their own words. The researcher developed themes from the responses. In question 1, all of the familial caregivers indicated that their recruitment into caregiving was necessitated by familial duty and was not a choice. Everyone interviewed spoke of a sense of duty or an obligation.

These sentiments are perhaps best demonstrated by this statement from family caregiver Interviewee 1, who said when asked why he didn't just walk away and let someone else take care of his mother,

"I guess a sense of obligation, a sense of family."

Familial caregiver #2 stated,

"There was no one else to do it. I was thrust into it. My other siblings —I don't know if you want to say lost interest or just chose not to be participatory."

These feelings of duty are contrasted with those of Interviewee 5, the professional caregiver, who said,

"It was because of circumstances," and further explained how watching his father a surgeon, "improve the health and quality of living of a lot of his patients" had significantly influenced his decision. Interviewee 5 went on to reiterate that he "...thought it would be a good thing for me to follow in his footsteps."

There were significant differences between the professional and familial caregivers responses to question one. The family caregivers had not chosen this career path or role, but instead it had been foisted upon them. Conversely, the professionals had decided this was what they wanted to do with their life. The interviews with the familial caregivers had a common theme of frustration. They often articulated that many of their hopes and dreams had been usurped by these traumatic events. However, they unanimously voiced that they wished they could do more to help their loved one. professional female Interviewee six stated,

"I think my self-esteem suffered on many levels because I was unable to concentrate on my career choices and I was unable to change the outcome for the patient. I think I did pretty much everything I could, given the situation. But, then what have I actually accomplished?"

<u>Interview Question 2.</u> How has this positively or negatively impacted your life?

The responses to question 2 on the life impact of caregiving were diverse and ranging. The familial responses were stronger and seemed to convey disruption in their plans and lives. Whereas, the professional caregivers had chosen caregiving as their careers and were achieving their goals.

Family participant 1, said,

"I think in a positive way it's made me more resilient. Maybe I'm able to look at things in a different way"

Another family participant stated,

"From a negative perspective, physically you get very tired."

A positive response from family caregiver 8,

"The medical regime keeps me going and from being overly emotional because there are certain things that need to be done, appointments or blood or whatever. If your doing these things you think there is hope. It is good to have something to focus on and hold on to."

Familial female caregiver 2 said,

"The medical options were like an anchor. You depend so much on the medical advice to direct you. You say, he knows something I don't know and when he suggests something you say let's run with this. I just read and read-any thing I could get my hands on about the diagnosis."

Family participant 1 agreed,

"It really helped me that I was really in the present. I partialize and don't look to far down the road and that helps me to cope better."

Another participant mentioned this as well; family respondent 4

said,

"You have to partialize, you have to focus on what's going on. As I said earlier, live in the present every day by day, and stay there and just share the love and share your feelings and your beliefs with that person to try to feed them as much positive energy as you can, hoping that that will make a difference."

Although, Interviewee 8 stated,

"A real negative for me, was that I tended to over-eat because I was tired all the time and I needed the energy. At the time it didn't seem important if I gained a couple of pounds but then it just kept going on and soon it was fifty pounds. It was a coping mechanism. Somehow in the moment, you aren't as important as the patient."

The professional respondents mentioned how much extra work they had to do but this question was best summarized by professional Interviewee 3, who stated,

" I don't believe that I necessarily gained a whole lot. I mean, the memories were good, and the frustration wasn't so bad that I feel that that was the prominent factor."

Another male professional commented,

"This is what I've always wanted to do. Sure it is hard but how many people get to get up everyday and do what they love?"

Professional caregiver #3 stated,

"It is easier for me to be a caregiver at work and then come home and recharge. When I deal with a patent at work I deal with the issues at hand and then I close the book on the case. At the end of the day I can deal with my own family, personal life and that is something you learn to do because it is necessary to recharge, over many years. But when your family member is there all the time, you of course cannot close the page or chapter. You have to continue with it day and day and day."

<u>Interview Question 3.</u> Did you have doubts about your ability or willingness to take on this role?

None of the respondents indicated that they had any real doubts about their ability to perform caretaking tasks. However, the familial caregivers expressed more trepidition. This was a new arena and they were concerned they did not have enough medical knowledge for the periods of caregiving at home. They expressed that the responsibility was daunting. The nearest to that sentiment was familial caregiver 2, who said that she had,

"…there are moments of being afraid that you won't do as good a job as you should." In contrast, she went on to say, "No…you should be able to do it."

Familial caregiver #1 said,

I didn't have the luxury of deciding whether to care for her or not. There was no one else I had to."

However professional caregiver #5,

"I didn't have any doubts about my ability to take on the role but, I wasn't sure I was willing to commit indefinetly. I knew my work would be impacted negatively and I had to find a balance between my needs and the patient."

Professional caregiver #3 shared that sentiment,

"It is very different when it is your family duty versus your job. As a physician, I can quit any time I want but family caregivers don't always have that option.

Professional caregiver #7 stated,

"I was trained in medicine for seven years and am confident in my abilities. But, I can't imagine being an emotionally distressed family caregiver and faced with having to digest the medical venacular and options cold turkey."

This implied a sense of competency in each respondent.

The willingness of all participants to perform the caretaking tasks is also noteworthy. However, from a gender perspective, two male respondents indicated they either wanted to "walk away," as professional 7 indicated, or that they sometimes did abandon the duty, as familial respondent 3 did. None of the female respondents expressed a desire to walk away. Male, Interviewee 3 stated,

> "The timing of it was variable. Sometimes I was thrust into a very difficult period and other times there was less—and other times the frustration level led to sometimes abandoning the duty. At one period in my brothers illness, it was so hard to deal with that I had to get away. It was a survival mechanism of sorts. My mother's illness was an extended period of care, which resulted in a significant degree of pain, but I was able to push through it and keep working at it."

<u>Interview Question 4.</u> What qualities are perceived to be the most important for adaptation and endurance?

In responding to this question, each cargiver indicated that a break from caregiving duties was paramount. The break was important to both groups of caretakers. They all cited a need for time to interact with other people away from the patient as "more or less a survival mechanism."

In the words of professional Interviewee 7,

…is a need for a distraction, be it shopping, meditation, exercise, or eating, something to take their mind away from the daily pain they had to witness.

Familial caregiver #4 said,

"You have to step back and take a break. It is hard when the patient needs you twenty-four seven, but you have to get away or you can't keep going."

Female familial caregiver #2 reported,

"Well, you take little naps and you eat however…it's a little destructive, but it gets you there."

Several of the respondents also indicated the importance of the routine imposed by the medical profession. That routine with its little goals to be achieved gave the respondents a sense of power when they could see small achievements being accomplished.

Familial caregiver 6 said,

"But you feel that you're participating and you are helping. Maybe you're not, but you feel that way." Once again, the medical regimen kept the end goal in sight."

Familial caregiver #8,

"It helped me a lot to know that the professionals taking care of my son cared and I took great comfort in the information they gave me or the explanations and procedures they had. I felt like it was a team and I wasn't in it alone and it lessened the burden."

Interviewee 5 said of being a physician and a caregiver,

"The medical background helps provide structure and a objective. When you to understand the difficulties of physical and emotional well-being not only in the patient, but in yourself. Often you would want to intervene medically in a way in which you're not supposed to. But, that's because you want to do something and there's a sense of frustration that would make you want to help the loved one. Also, I think with some background you have a good idea of what's going on, sometimes more than the other medical personal and family."

Denial appeared to be a coping device for familial caregivers more than professional caregivers. Family caregiver 8 indicated that denial was a powerful coping mechanism for her, because to her,

"If you're convinced that at the end of the road, no matter what I'm doing, he's going to die, then you can stop right there."

Family caregiver #2 lamented,

"If you don't have hope, you can't get up each day and you have to for the patient."

The medical practice regimen appeared to a provide structure and hope to the caregivers. One 46-year-old female caregiver said of her dying brother,

"Even when you know it is hopeless, you keep searching because if you don't, then you have to accept that the patient will die and that is unbearable."

It also, appeared that hope was just as important to enable both groups of caregivers to cope with the hardships associated with caregiving. The two traits are basically the opposite sides of the same coin. Whether hope is putting faith in God, as Interviewee 1 indicated, or whether "it's just foolish hope," as expressed by Interviewee 2, hope plays a big part in all caregivers' ability to adapt and endure. This issue is discussed further in question 8.

<u>Interview Question 5.</u>   In retrospect, would you do anything differently to balance the care for the patient and the care for yourself?

The caregivers all expressed a desire to have changed at least some

aspect of their prior caregiving experience. Female, family caregiver

#2 wished she had tried to

"…format it a little bit better, tried to map it out better, in order to try to structure it (caregiving)."

While female familial respondent # 2 thought,

"You hit the wall if you don't take a break. Because your so entrenched it can be difficult to step away……you have to be aware. It's tough but you have to be aware of yourself too. I don't mean go out on the town, but maybe just a nap or a bubble bath-but you need to take a breather."

In contrast, professional caregiver Interviewee 3 said that his,

"…biggest recollection of sadness and things is that the frustration level, sometimes the impatience that you would show as a family caretaker, was such that you look back and wish you could have relived those moments and prevented them from happening or tried to be more patient."

Basically, as professional respondent #1 said, "Hindsight is 20/20."

Trauma surgeon #7 said,

" I mean, I don't know I exercise and work out. I try to stay busy and am active in the community, and stuff like that. I don't know that I do anything "specifically" to take care of myself. I just try to keep some balance, but it isn't easy."

Each group stressed the need for time away from the patient.

They felt that burnout was inevitable if the caregiver needs were muted. However, it was evident that the professional caregivers appeared to have more balanced lives, between caregiving and personal needs and interests.

<u>Interview Question 6.</u> Has your ability to interact with others in relationships or your social connectedness been impacted by this caregiving experience?

There was no consensus to this question. Familial interviewee #1 said,

"…that he wasn't affected on the surface but that I put up more walls with people and had few close friends."

Familial caregiver Interviewee 8 said,

"I that I have few friends that understood my reasons for not wanting to go out when I am invited."

Professional participant #3 reports in his caregiving experience,

"So, I think that I was held back for awhile and whether that would have happened naturally or not, I don't know. But, caregiving does change the way you react socially to those around you when you're caring for a loved one."

Male Professional caregiver #5 commented,

"I can't really enjoy my friends as much as before…I think I probably am depressed and should go talk to someone.

It is just that it would be so painful to talk about everything that has happened. I just can't motivate myself."

The interviewees' social lives in both groups are affected by the caregiving experience and isolation is a discernible trend. The family members worlds' became focused on the ill family member to the detriment of the caregiver needs. The professionals seemed to report that there social lives diminished because of the grueling work schedule. Although, professional caregiver #5 appears to have a clinical depression. Perhaps due to his unwillingness to process the sad and difficult elements of his career. The professionals may perceive emotional investment in their patients as unprofessional or not doing their job.

<u>Interview Question 7.</u> How do you feel this experience has impacted your ability to enjoy and progress in other areas of your life?

This question also got a mixed response. Familial interviewees caregivers #1 and #6 both indicated how much they had learned to mute their feelings and how they did not really feel high highs or low lows.

A male familial respondent stated,

"I have numbed myself to disappointment."

A male, familial subject said,

"I think there is a piece of me that keeps walls up because I am fearful of getting into this situation again. The less people in your sphere that depend on you the less chance you have of getting pulled in again. Although I know that is not a good way to think, I can't help it."

Another collective negative risk factor for the participants was that future goals and plans were changed forever. A 52-year-old nurse and family caregiver said,

"You can never get that time back. You feel derailed. It affects my motivation because I never know if I'll be able to follow through on something because of her changing condition."

Professional caregiver #7 felt,

"...things don't seem as fun as they should."

This contrasted with the other interviewees who said that they had gained from the experience.

Female familial caregiver # 4 stated,

"That is an interesting question actually, with reference to my state, because I don't think that I even considered that." She said that she had "…gained more self-esteem in the fact that I became even more in control of whether it was my life, my ideas, my—whatever I did."

Professional caregiver # 3

"…I was relatively restricted in my social sphere, and doing very little in the way of outside activities with multiple groups of people…I became very active and have become even more outgoing since that time."

Clearly, the aftermath of a family caregiving experience seems to influence people, but the multiple variables unique to each situation make it difficult to tell how someone is going to be affected. The professional and familial groups each reported negative and positive inluences on their lives from the caregiving experiences.

Interview Question 8. Have hope and spirituality been factors in your ability to cope and endure throughout this experience?

Hope played a significant role in the familial respondent's ability to cope with the caregiving experience. The familial caregivers agreed that hope or a belief in a higher power were a source of strength and resilience.

The mother of a young boy in a persistant neuro-vegetative state, said it best:

"Accepting it is not possible."

Another familial caregiver said,

"you have to be thinking,-no, we can beat this. Otherwise why try?"

Familial caregiver interviewee 8 felt that,

"God could heal anybody if He chose, for whatever reason." She went on to say, "…you have to have faith in God, and faith that even though you don't understand the circumstance, He's in control."

Professional caregiver # 4 stated,

"Because of what happened, I became more spiritual, so that for me I would find strength by believing in an afterlife, also, by believing in different things of a new age perspective. I began to search for a meaning in what had happened and I read books on spiritualism of every kind."

In contrast professional interviewee #3 felt,

"As a physician you realize that life is precious and temporary, and there will be a time when your loved one is gone. Whether that is met with relief due to the pain or suffering, or whether it is a cause for sadness I think spirituality is important. I believe there is a purpose for our lives and for others' lives and the interactions between them."

Another male professional caregiver #7 stated,

"As a physician I am very pragmatic and rely less on spirituality or hope. It is based on what you see day to day in your work, in terms of illness and people dying and people suffering, so that you understand that those things are transient, they change. Sometimes it may take many months or years but they do change. And you know there are periods where situations improve and then deteriorate but, eventually they all pass."

All familial interviewees said that spirituality was important in helping them to cope and endure, but none gave it the same prominence as familial caregivers Interviewees 1 and 8. Overriding or "simple hope" provided each respondent with an inner strength to keep going. Spirituality also played an important part in all the participants' ability to cope but was more important to some than to others. However, the professional caregivers relied less on spirituality as a facor for coping. They were more pragmatic and less emotional regarding their caregiving experience.

Analysis of Qualitative Self-Report Questionnaire Results

This section provides analyses of the responses to the qualitative questionnaire that was administered to familial and professional caregivers. Control participants were not given this questionaire.

To explore more about the reasons for the development of PTSD in familial and professional caregivers, the participants n = 40 completed a 6-question qualitative follow-up questionnaire (Appendix E). Participants were allowed to check off as many responses as they wanted. The questions are below. Following each question is a table, Tables 18 through 23, which provides response and frequency data for the follow-up questions.

<u>Analysis of Qualitative Self-Report Questionnaire Results</u>

Question 1: What inspired or challenged you to become a caregiver?

Table 18

<u>Frequency of Caregiver Answers for Question 1</u>

Response	Familial Caregivers		Professional Caregivers	
	Freq.	%	Freq.	%
1 Role model/mentor	0	0	1	5
2 Sense of fulfillment	0	0	7	35
3 Care for a family member	17	85	2	10
4 Compassion	3	15	5	25
5 Competency/Good at it	0	0	5	25

Note:.N=40

Question 2: What are the qualities that have enabled you to adapt,

endure and maintain your sense of resilience?

Table 19

<u>Frequency of Caregiver Answers for Question 2</u>

Response	Familial Caregivers		Professional Caregivers	
	Freq.	%	Freq.	%
Support of others	2	10	3	15
Compassion	2	10	9	45
Keeping things in perpestive	1	5	3	15
Spirituality	8	40	1	5
Competency and skill	7	35	4	20

N=40

Question 3: How has caregiving positively affected your life?

Table 20

<u>Frequency of Caregiver Answers for Question 3</u>

Response	Familial Caregivers		Professional Caregivers	
	Freq.	%	Freq.	%
Making a difference	7	35	13	65
Helping others	5	25	1	5
Challenge	1	5	2	10
Keeping close to family	7	35	3	20

Note: N=40

Question 4: How has caregiving negatively affected your life?

Table 21

<u>Frequency of Caregiver Answers for Question 4</u>

Response	Familial Caregivers		Professional Caregivers	
	Freq.	%	Freq.	%
Exhaustion	15	35	1	5
Stress	4	20	1	5
Feeling overwhelmed	1	5	7	35

Response	Familial Caregivers		Professional Caregivers	
	Freq.	%	Freq.	%
Sadness	1	5	2	10
Long hours	11	9	9	45

Note: N=40

Question 5: What surprising thing did you learn about yourself?

Table 22

<u>Frequency of Caregiver Answers for Question 5</u>

Response	Familial Caregivers		Professional Caregivers	
	Freq.	%	Freq.	%
Spirituality	3	15	1	5.00
Burn out	0	0	1	5.00
Level of caring	12	60	7	35.00
Ability to distance emotionally	5	25	11	55.00

Note: N=40

Question 6: What coping mechanism would you recommend to other

caregivers?

Table 23

Frequency of Caregiver Answers for Question 6

	Familial Caregivers		Professional Caregivers	
Response	Freq.	%	Freq.	%
Social supports	4	20	6	30
Sense of humor	2	10	1	5
Time for self	0	0	3	15
Persistence	1	5	4	20
Control of emotions	0	0	2	10
Spirituality	13	65	4	20

Note: N=40

From the results, inspiration (question 1) appears essential for both kinds of caregivers, though their inspirational sources were different. For familial caregivers, the care for a family member was the main source (85%; see Table 18); on the contrary, a sense of fulfillment was the main source for professional caregivers (35%). Consistent with the previous analyses, resiliency seems to have little effect on PTSD scores for either control or familial group of caregivers and does have an effect on professional caregivers.

On the other hand, it is understandable that the negative influences of caregiving (question 4, long hours, 65% in family group and 45% in professional group; Table 21), seem to be correlated to PTSD scores for familial caregivers (one-sided p value = 0.07. Negative influences might also affect the PTSD tendency for professional caregivers (p value = 0.1150). Long hours are generally necessary to take care of trauma patients. This is a challenge that caregivers of trauma patients have to face.

The negative influences of caregiving on the participants' lives (question 4) affected the tendency to acquire PTSD for professional caregivers and might also affect family caregivers. Table 20 also shows that 65% of the professional group and 35% of family group said caregiving allowed them to make a difference in the world. Another 35% of the family group said that caregiving kept them closer to their families.

The methods for coping with PTSD appear to affect professional caregivers only. Of the professionals, 30% said that seeking social support was a good method to decrease the possibility of PTSD. Another 20% said that persistence or spirituality helped them to cope with the signs of PTSD. Methods for coping with the pressure and decreasing the possibility of acquiring PTSD still need further study.

Chapter 5

Discussion

<u>Summary and Interpretation of Findings</u>

The results of this study were consistent with the goal to gain an understanding of the impact of caregiving for a trauma patient. An exploration of the adaptive process and protective risk factors enhance our ability to assist those in need. The data from the quantitative study indicates a association between the independent and dependent variables for the sample population. The findings from the qualitative interview shed light on the emotional toll of the experience on caregivers. Their interpretation of their role provides more data for in-depth analyses to provide an understanding of the difficulties inherent in the role of caregiver from a professional or familial perspective.

This section also discusses the standardized instruments findings and research questions, as well as, the qualitative interviews and hypothesis. The following section provides a detailed summary of the findings for the independent/dependent variables in the study and examines those results as compared to other studies in this area.

Hypothesis 1

"There will be significant differences on PTSD scores in familial and professional caregiver compared to control participants consistent with secondary traumatization."

The results of this study support the hypothesis that professional and familial caregivers experience secondary traumatization from their contact with the trauma patient. These results support the findings by Stamm (1999) regarding those who have been traumatized without actually experiencing the trauma firsthand. The caregivers reported commonalities in the symptoms based on the uniqueness of their experience and perceptions. These findings confirm previous research in the literature review by Hawley & Dehaan (1996), Lindemann (1944), Walsh (1996) and Wollen & Wollen (1993), and Rutter (1993) and their studies on secondary responses to trauma. The most frequently reported symptoms were emotional sadness, sleep disturbance, increased startle response, and avoidant thoughts.

All participants remarked that their life goals and plans had been unexpectedly disrupted. They expressed concern that their needs had been muted in an effort to care for the patient. The caregivers had a sense that their immediate needs were not as important as those of their patient. Over time this created additional wounds and lowered self-esteem for the caregiver. This loss of control in one's life goes to the very core of PTSD and exacerbates the caregiver symptoms.

Hypothesis 2

"There is an inverse relationship, between the two measures of resiliency and PTSD."

This study showed a negative correlation between Post Traumatic Stress Disorder symptoms and resiliency scores for familial caregivers. As the symptoms of PTSD grew higher the resiliency scores were lower. Resiliency, which is construed as an intellectual component, allows us to cope, renew, and reorganize during and after a traumatic episode. The fact that familial caregivers have low resiliency scores and high PTSD scores is possibly due to the fact that they muted their feelings in an effort to maintain functionality in the midst of shattered hopes and disrupted lives, as described by Rutter (1993). The family participants emphatically stated that "falling apart was not an option because I needed to be able to take care of the patient." There was a consensus that attending to one's own needs and grieving later was the efficient thing to do. Perhaps this internalization of emotions resulted in lower resiliency scores because the familial caregiver was not renewed by outside sources and continually depleted their reserves. In fact, the test results showed that the family caregivers had the highest PTSD scores of the three groups and the lowest resiliency scores. The family participants perceived "resiliency" as maturity and self-discipline that was learned through experience and role models. The relationship between resiliency and secondary PTSD symptoms in controls can be explained by control participants not having to deal with trauma patients every day, so their resiliency comes from other sources. Therefore this group reported low PTSD scores and high resiliency scores.

On the other hand, professional caregivers results showed the lower the PTSD score the higher the resiliency score. The professional caregivers do not have to be as guarded and restrictive of their emotions as the familial caregivers. Professionals can be aware of their emotions and explore without fear of being totally overwhelmed. Messner (1993), describes this as "cognition over emotion and being aware of what you are feeling in the moment." (p.128). The seem to be able to balance all areas in their life and restore and replenish their energy.

<u>Hypothesis 3</u>

"There will be gender effects on familial and professional caregivers PTSD scores."

Differences on the basis of gender were less pronounced than expected. The quantitative measures showed only a marginal increase in PTSD scores for female professional caregivers. This could result from an increased emotional response to the trauma patient's distress with a lack of processing the emotional response. The female professional caregivers reported a higher incidence of multiple somatic complaints, which suggested internalization and repression of her feelings.

There was no significant differences reported amongst familial caregivers as relates to gender. The family caregiver group was surprising, because the sample of

n = 20 produced a group of 14 males and 6 females. It would have seemed that the majority of familial caretakers would have been women. One of the unexpected findings was that the majority of the caregivers were men and that they were taking care of patients at home. This makes it more difficult to rely on suppositions regarding gender attitudes and emotions. Both the men and women in this familial group were insightful and articulate. This familial caregiver group produced gender neutral results from the quantitative and qualitative measures. The only notable exception was that the male respondents had debated walking away from their situation. The women never mentioned that as an option. These results support the findings in the literature review by Seelbach (1977), that women have a stronger sense of familial responsibility, "emphasizing duty, protection, and care." The qualitative aspect to the research adds another dimension of richness and depth. One notable point from the researcher's perspective surfaced when the familial and professional groups were taking the qualitative semi-structured interviews. The female participants were often tearful and emotive when speaking about the patient. They appeared to want to talk in great length about what had happened. In contrast, the men were more factual than emotional and resisted becoming overly expressive.

Research Questions

Research Question 1

What are the experiences of secondary traumatization in professional and familial caregivers and what are the major difficulties of these experiences?

This study has established a correlation between PTSD symptoms and familial and professional caregiver participants and by analyzing the symptoms of PTSD that the participants described. The symptoms exemplify the struggles that the caregivers undertake. Although, a number of the interviewees stated that they would "do it all over again," their pain was apparent. Another common theme was, "You feel like you're in it alone, and the isolation is difficult."

A 40-year-old surgeon had a different perspective that resulted from his professional ability to distance himself emotionally. He stated,

> "My chief told me in residency that you do the best you can and if the patient dies you move on and see the next patient. The clock keeps ticking, and there is always another patient."

This surgeon said he was desensitized and immune to the emotional havoc that suffering and death can inflict on caregivers. Yet he scored 19 on the PTSD symptom scale. One wonders whether his affect and bravado are caused by conscious or unconscious factors.

A common complaint found among the qualitative interviewees was exhaustion. Family members were especially overwhelmed by the limited support of helpers and their resultant sleep deprivation. Compassion fatigue and burnout were prevalent in almost all cases. Yet, every participant stated they would do it again.

One 33-year-old family caregiver who had lovingly cared for her mother for years until her death, tearfully said,

"It was horrible but I would give anything to be able to do it again today."

Research Question 2

What is the nature of risk factors that aggravate, or protective factors that help to eliminate the difficulties of the caretaking experience?

The discussion of what the professional and familial participants recommend for protective risk factors that will enable others in their position to sustain and triumph over adversity follows. The caregivers who appeared to be the highest functioning and with the lowest symptoms of PTSD appeared to have found some strength to keep them going. This study found four prevalent protective factors: social connectedness, spirituality, self-confidence and resiliency. Resiliency has already been addressed; the discussion below addresses the other three factors. The results from the qualitative interview sheds light on key protective factors as displayed in tables18-23 in the results chapter. Clearly, social supports are important for the caregivers to maintain a balance between the caregiving role and everyday life as Fink (1995) discusses in her theoretical model, "of the three types of resources for caregivers, the primary feature is social connectedness" (p. 139). A social support network can validate the caregiver's fears, help to alleviate worries, and provide a valuable respite and enjoyable escape from patient duties.

Most caregivers reported feeling isolated and "in it alone." They became myopically focused on their caregiving role and allowed their world to become smaller and smaller. This lack of support and interaction with the outside world is very detrimental to the caregiver.

One female family caregiver stated,

"It wasn't that I didn't have time to see friends, I just couldn't sit with them and talk about mundane things while he was home so ill."

Some caregivers have limited backup and relief to help them take care of family members. Familial caregivers felt that the longer the caregiving role, the more isolated life became, which led to despair. The studies by Hamburg and Killilea (1985) and Edelstein (1988) support the finding that social support for the caregiver is a key factor to sucessful coping. Social connectedness is one of the most important variables in the study of caregivers and resiliency. We may examine social interactions using tools such as Social Network Assessements that provide us with insight into the coping mechanisms of caregivers. "Concepts of love, trust, kindness, caring, sharing, giving, receiving, influencing, teaching, belonging and relating are important parts of the human condition that can be studied, nurtured or appreciated by examining an individual's connections to others" (Pilisuk & Wong, 2001). The maintenance of social connectedness can promote open and realistic communication in a caring, empathic environment. This is delineated by Medalie (1985), "Social support has a mediating effect that stimulates the development of coping strategies and promotes mastery." (p. 534). It appears that social connections and support are pivotal to maintaining psychological well-being.

Further, a sense of confidence enabled the caregiver to continue. High self-esteem and mastery of skills seemed to be a protective factor that aided both the professional and familial caregivers in this study as noted in the findings of Kadner (1989), that "adequate ego strength increases the likelihood of resilience to adversity" (p. 20). Self-confidence armed the caregiver with the hardiness and buoyancy to care for the patient over an extended period of time. The professionals reported that emotional distance was an effective coping method. Whereas, familial caregivers felt that the task of the medical regimen and researching resources and options were anchors in the caregiving battle. This competency and resourcefulness helped the caregivers to feel empowered and strengthened their resolve to prevail. Also, past accomplishments can provide experiences to draw upon during times of adversity. Children have a more difficult time with grief and resiliency because they have less life experience from which to draw, which is supported by studies by Wollen and Wollen (1995), and O'Grady and Metz (1987).

In essence self-confidence allows the caregiver to have a sense of control amidst the chaos of a traumatic episode. These findings are supported by the studies of Flannery (1986), Lewis, Gottesman and Gutstein (1979), Gottesman and Lewis (1982), Pollack (1979), and Fink (1995).

One of the risk factors that can aggravate the caretaking experience is a sense of guilt. One 41-year-old, male, professional caregiver who had cared for his acutely ill mother for decades stated,

> "Even after all the dedication and love, you always feel you could do more. I concentrated on my mother's care because I was the only one and I couldn't abandon her. So, I am developmentally delayed for my age, no children, career kind of stuck, and still the guilt is always there."

Research Question 3

What part do spirituality and hope play in resiliency for caregivers?

It appears that the caregivers who maintained a sense of spirituality or a meaning behind the event were able to cope better. These participants displayed signs of withdrawal, anger, and helplessness. Spirituality and hope appeared to be significant protective factors amongst the caregiver respondents. The most common finding, regarding spirituality was the importance of finding a meaning in the experience. The caregivers drew strength from their faith that there was a reason for the episode and this supports the articles in the literature review regarding hope and spirituality as key factors in resiliency by Lindsay (1992), Oe (1977), Barnard (2000), and Seigel (1986).

Spirituality had different connotations for the caregiver participants: some observed in a formal religion, a number engaged in mystical practice, while others believed in a higher power or order. There were no agnostics among the participants. The sense of an ultimate purpose appeared to give caregivers hope and sustenance to bear the palpable grief of pain and death.

174

A 41-year-old familial caregiver stated,

"If you maintain a feeling that there is a master plan or a reason that this has happened, it provides a source of strength. I don't know what I would do without my belief system. I pray all the time and it gets me through."

Spirituality and hope may provide a buffer for most caregivers. A 47-year-old physician reported,

"Sometimes when the patient and I know that he is going to die, I just sit with him while he prays, and somehow it helps me too."

These reports support the findings of Haley and Dehan, (1996) and their observation that spirituality allows caregivers to maintain a belief and hope for the future. Some professional caregivers stated that the rewards of caregiving were the primary motivation for their choice of career paths. The spiritual care of and service to others can bring fulfillment and meaning into one's life. The consensus among the caregivers was that spirituality and hope made survival feasible.

Research Question 4

What do professional and familial caregivers recommend to others to help them sustain the caregiving battle?

When asked in question 6 of Appendix E, "What protective factors do you recommend for other caregivers?" the collective answer for both groups seemed to be moderation and a balance between the needs of the patient and their own personal needs. The main suggestion for the familial caretaker was maintaining a social network. The benefits of this are twofold: it allows the caregiver to vent frustrations and fears, and gives the caretaker time to escape and enjoy other interests. Even something as inconsequential as working out helped the caregiver (also recommended by professional caregivers) to take time for themselves, work off frustrations, and process events.

Some professional respondents recommended maintaining a sense of humor. One emergency room trauma nurse who had been in that occupation for more than 33 years said,

"If people heard the staff joking, they probably wouldn't understand, but it keeps us going at work and it keeps us connected as a team and ultimately results in better care for the patient."

However, a number of professional caregivers noted that allowing yourself to care about the patient, while mainitaining a professional distance was a key factor for resiliency. A 37-year-old male child psychiatrist discussed the thing he learned about himself that surprised him, when he openly stated,

"I always thought of myself as really self-centered, which was okay with me, but I was amazed to find out how much I cared about these people. I really like them and they matter to me."

Yet he reports a balanced life full of personal interests and activities. Clearly, it is much easier for the professional to find a healthy balance than the familial caregiver.

Impact on Dependent Variable

PTSD

The first quantitative test the Modified PTSD Symptom Scale indicated positive findings. The sample population completed this self-report questionaire to discern whether caregivers of trauma patients showed symptoms of secondary traumatization. The findings were significant in respect to symptomatology. The highest score for vicarious traumatization was the family caregivers with a mean score of 24.15. Each respondent in this group reported signs of PTSD for a lengthy period of time. The highest scoring symptom was feeling emotionally labile and very easily upset. The participants also complained of irritability and difficulty concentrating. They experienced intrusive thoughts and reported difficulty with their startle response. Family participants had increased hypervigilance and were unable to disrupt this high alert status and relax. The majority of family caregivers felt an extreme sense of isolation due to limited social supports. The number one factor upon which they all agreed was that their future plans had been disrupted irrevocably by the sudden trauma inculcated into their lives. These findings support the studies of Van Der Kolk (1996), Hermann (1992,) Perry (1999) and their array of symptoms related to trauma response.

The professional caregivers scores were noteworthy on the PTSD Scale. However, this group scored a bit lower than the familial caregivers for symptoms of PTSD. Therefore, the results of this quantitative test indicate that both groups of caregivers exhibited signs of secondary traumatization. The professionals observed similar symptoms of feeling emotionally upset and reported sleep disturbance. Another interesting finding for the professional was that they noted experiencing physical and somatic complaints related to the stressors of caregiving. This could be due to their hectic schedules and not taking the time to address their feelings as described by Messner's (1993) findings on resident physicians and resiliency characteristics. The number one symptom reported among professional caregivers was intrusive thoughts. They found it difficult to totally dismiss some specific, difficult patient cases even with their professional emotional distance.

The 20-member control group took the PTSD Scale. The participants consisted of 11 females and 9 males. The results were minimal as expected with a mean score of 7.10. The results for the normal population without PTSD symptomatology is less than 5. It is of note that the PTSD scores for the control group were mildly higher than those found in the published studies, possibly because this study began one month after the September 11th, 2002, attacks on the World Trade Center. At that time, people were generally more distressed than previously and most likely served to mildly elevate the scores. However, the results were in the borderline normal high range and were not significant enough to impact the results of the study. The control group was experiencing slightly increased hypervigilance and irritability as well as difficulty concentrating. Also, the control group commonly experienced avoidant or repressive thoughts, preferring to push incoming information away rather than process it.

<u>Impact of Predictor Variables</u>

<u>Resiliency</u>

The correlation between resiliency and PTSD is perhaps surprising. According to the Pearson test, resiliency has no effect on the PTSD symptom scores in controls or familial caregivers as the p value for the null hypothesis are 0.38 and 0.20 respectively, much larger than 0.10. Therefore it is not possible to reject the null hypothesis. However, in professional caregivers, there is a negative correlation between resiliency and PTSD scores, with a coefficient = -0.35.

Therefore, when the familial caregivers take care of family members, emotion plays a much more important role than resiliency. The resiliency influence cannot impact as strongly. In contrast, the professionals do not have as much emotional involvement, so resiliency becomes a factor. Therefore, there is a negative correlation within familiy caregivers; the higher the symptoms of PTSD, the lower the resiliency score.

A lack of resiliency leaves the caregiver raw and vulnerable to their emotions. Maturity evokes a more thoughtful and controlled response that can generate endurance and survival. One female family caregiver stated, "If you are a healthy being and you are in an emotionally difficult situation, then you have to intellectualize your emotions to function. There is time to indulge in sadness later." It is important, however, to note that active processing and reflection is a necessary and important component to growth. Unfortunately, the familial caregiver does not appear to restore their resiliency from outside sources, and focuses instead on their patient.

Both professional and familial groups felt that role models and mentors had instilled in them a sense of resiliency and that endurance and survival were possible as described by the studies of Ursano (1995), Kadner (1989) and Hamilton, McCubbin, Thompson, & Allen (1997).

Susan Cooney, Ph.D.

The protective factors that contribute to resiliency appear to be intellectual awareness and external environment controls such as social networks that aid in coping with adversity and alleviating emotional pain as observed by the research of Kobasa (1979), Leske & Jiricka (1998), and Montgomery, Gonyea & Hooynan (1985).

The findings in this study, found a link between protective factors and secondary traumatic response in caregivers, that corresponds to the literature review findings by Ursano 1973), Holaday & Merrill (1994), Nolan (1992) and Weiss (1988). These studies all address the difficulty of caregiving for patients following traumatic episodes and the common protective factors have been reported. These factors can help to nourish future caregivers during difficult periods as described by Gottesman and Lewis (1982). The stress on the caregivers of a patient suffering from disability and illness can result in increased levels of frustration, a loss of control of one's own personal life, and a heavy burden of sadness. If people also vary in resiliency, the question arises, can resiliency be learned? Can we foster some protective factors to enable individuals and families to persist under great duress? Hopefully, future studies in this area will provide much needed answers.

Limitations and Delimitations

This research attempts to clarify that secondary traumatization may be identified and elucidates a characteristic symptom picture of coping mechanisms. Some issues jeopardize the internal and external validity of this study. The participants were voluntary and were specifically involved in at least four years caregiving following a traumatic episode. Their exposure to a wide variety of traumatic episodes generalize the findings. The small size of the sample and the method of sampling creates a further threat to the validity of the research project, because it selects volunteers from a certain context ie; trauma facilities in the New York and Massachusetts area. Therefore, inference can only be made to the exact population and description given. Of the 60 participants, 32 had been or were in therapy during the study. The World Trade Center attacks on September 11th contributed to a generally heightened sense of stress, but did not significantly impact the results of this study. This possible conjoint therapy of more than 52% percent partaking in outside counseling could create a bias. Another consideration is that the participants were in different stages of grief and mental health, which makes comparisons more difficult and this snapshot may create a significant bias. There is a risk of the Hawthorne effect wherein participants realize they are in a study and this impacts their statements of attitude. The self-report tests are subject to social bias because the participants may adjust their statements to please the researchr or the participants' desire to present themselves in a favorable light. Internal validity is threatened by history, selection, and maturation. The study does not include specific religious affiliations, all levels of socioeconomic backgrounds, or ethnic diversity.

There are limitations in the instruments, by using quantitative methods to report on subtle human experiences. The qualitative interviews provide a rich tapestry of unique information. However, the subject may be self-conscious about revealing things to the researcher, whereas, the qualitative questionaires allowed the patients to be more disinhibited and report their results anonomously. There is always the risk of researcher bias in recording and interpreting the data. Also, there is the risk that the patient is unconsciously aware of what he is feeling, perhaps too afraid to explore his emotions. There was no observable increase in level of distress reported from the study by participants in any of the three groups.

Implications for Future Research

This is an important area for future research because additional findings may help past and future caregivers of victims of traumatic episodes. Ideally, future studies would test pre/post-trauma scores in longitudinal studies of resiliency and PTSD. It appears that resiliency is a protective factor, consisting of self-discipline and control that may be learned from role-models or behavioral/cognitive approaches. Further studies on resiliency must continue to explore the emotional and intellectual responses of caregivers in different medical arenas. The researcher was interested in obtaining a conceptional and personal understanding of the participants' understanding and lived experience. The participant's attitudes, feelings, and behavioral changes throughout the process of caregiving are key to discovering protective factors. Additional research is needed to explore the links between secondary traumatization and the caregiver role to assess self-regulation and awareness. These findings will help increase the understanding of a poorly studied area and guard caregivers from burnout and compassion fatigue.

Eventually protective factors may be strengthened and risk factors prevented to enhance caregiver resiliency through greater examination of victim responses. Further exploration of dispositional resilience and hardiness are key to understanding their effect on familial and professional caregivers efforts to maintain physical and emotional health. It appears that resiliency scores decrease as additional strains are placed on the familial caregiver; this valuable information warrants further study. Future research could inform mental health and other professionals of strategies and methods to support the neglected needs of the caregivers of trauma. Scientists can provide a better understanding of the impact on the neuro-psychiatric components of the medial temporal lobe and amygdala. Unfortunately, the emotional effect and scarring from trauma has provided tangible evidence, as seen by magnetic resonance imaging.

Therefore the physical and emotional impact on the limbic system is forever. This study has demonstrated that secondary traumatization from the caregiver role may result in symptoms of Post Traumatic Stress Disorder and underscores the importance of preventative measures to assist caregivers in the struggle to sustain their role.

When we have a keener understanding of the coping and adaptation methods of the caregivers, we can gauge the efficacy of interventions and of treatment regimes. This information may help therapists and crisis teams to assess the nature and scope of the effects on caregivers and allow for better advocacy for therapeutic self-care and professional management plans. Longitudinal studies may advance the knowledge of protective factors and interventions for supporting the caregiver role. The findings from future studies in this area will help a multitude of people in various interpersonal stages of recovery such as, professional caregivers ie; physicians, firefighters, social workers, EMT's and familial caregivers of victims of chronic illness, sudden trauma and natural disasters maintain their caregiving capacity. The perception of objective and subjective burden as described by the participants helps to illuminate the different factors that can be controlled and alleviate the suffering of the caregiver. These findings support prior study results that social support, spirituality and hope are key factors for coping and endurance. National caregiver support groups and psychotherapy groups are becoming more common as caregivers search for help and strength to prevail. The burden of the caregiver is fraught with the emotional components of fear, guilt, exhaustion and sadness.

Grief reaction to trauma is explained in the seven stages by Elizabeth Kubler-

Ross, who states that ;

> Grief is a process of physical, emotional, social and cognitive reaction to loss.... People are like stained glass windows. They sparkle and shine when the sun is out, but when the darkness sets in their true beauty is revealed only if there is a light from within. (Kubler-Ross,1957 P. 28)

Future studies must learn from the valuable insights of the caregivers themselves. The privilege of their personal experiences and narratives are an invaluable tool for future investigations. Additional research may convince government officials to designate special budget allocations for additional expenditures to support the caregivers in the home. Some of these familial caregivers have had to take leave from there work indefinitely and are emotionally and monetarily facing difficult circumstances with limited resources. The National Family Caregiver Support Program has recently advocated for caregivers of elderly and disabled and in the state of Massachusetts and allocated $198,000.00 for The Long-term Care Ombudsman Program for 2002. That is a meager total amount for all the family caregivers in this state. Hopefully, future studies will demonstrate a need for caregiver relief and will increase this aid over time. Unfortunately, people are suffering today and recovery assistance is urgently needed for families to survive adversity. There is a silent epidemic in our society of anguished caregivers that has resulted in isolation, weariness and muted needs of the family member. We must urgently strive to empower and support this crisis with economic, therapeutic and social support, by continuing to study this important topic. Whether the conclusions in this study are specific or generic in nature they serve to provide a clearer understanding of the ordeal faced by the caregiver.

In Conclusion

This study has contributed to a better psychological understanding of the difficulties faced by caregivers in these groups. It is the personal hope of the researcher that the participants have benefited from a better insight into their motivations, perceptions, and feelings. Clearly, the caregiving role is awe-inspiring. The valor and strength of the human spirit and the willingness to provide support and tireless care in spite of an unknown outcome is wondrous. This human experience is laden with sacrifice, grief, and unexpected difficulties. This study has observed a wide range of individual responses and coping strategies and noted that successful caregivers of trauma may benefit from social connectedness, spirituality, self-confidence, and a sense of resiliency. The author suggests that these protective factors can be learned and achieved, resulting in optimal psychological health and functioning during the professional and familial caregivers' time of hardship. It is a noble and sacred mission to care for the needs of trauma patients.

"Wherever you find your role model, your inspiration or your motivation, you will discover that the essence of survival behavior is a reverence for all life and a compassionate response to all suffering" (Siegel, 1996, p. ix).

These participants graciously shared their caregiving experiences in an effort to further the study of secondary traumatization and resiliency factors, with the hope that the results of this study may contribute and enlighten future studies in this much needed area. More research is needed to explore links between secondary traumatization and the caregiver role and these findings may help us understand a poorly studied area and guard caregivers from burnout and emotional fatigue.

<u>References</u>

Astin, M.C., Lawrence, K., Foy, D; (1993). Post Traumatic Stress Disorder Among Battered Women. *Violence and Victims*, (1): 1728 Spring.

Atkins, R; Amenta, M; (1991). Family adaptation to AIDS: a comparative study. *Hospice Journal* 7 (1-2):71-83.

Barnard, David, (2000), *Crossing Over:Narratives of Palliative Care.* Oxford University Press.

Bloom, B. (1963). Definitional Aspects of the Crisis Concept, *Journal of Consulting Psychology,* 27, pp 498-502.

Borg, W.R., & Gall, M.D. (1989). *Educational Research.* New York: Longman.

Bowlby, J. (1969), *Attachment and Loss*, vol. 1 New York: Basic Books.

Bronfenbrenner, U. (1990). Discovering what families do. In D. Blankenhorne (Eds.), *Rebuilding the nest,* (pp 27-38) Milwaukee WI: Family Service of America.

Charney, D.S., Deutch, A.Y., Krystal, J.H, Southwick, S.M., (1993) Psychobilogic Mechanisms of Post Traumatic Stress Disorder, *Arch General Psychiatry*;50: 294-305.

Coyne, J.C. et al; (1990) Social Support, Interdependence and the Dilemmas of Helping in Sarason, S, Sarason, B. & Pierce, G.R. (Eds) *Social Support: an interactional* view (129-149), New York:Wiley.

Davis, M., (1993), Psychobiologic Mechanisms of PostTraumatic Stress Disorder. *Arch General Psychiatry*; 50:294-305.

Christianson, S.A. (1992). Emotional stress and eyewitness memory: A critical review. *Psychological Bulletin,* 112, 284-309.

Edelstein, Michael, (1988). Contaminated Communities: *The Psychosocial Effects of Residential Toxic Exposure*. Boulder: Westview Press.

Fife, Betsy; (1985). A model for predicting the adaptation of families to medical crisis: An analysis of role integration. *The journal of Nursing Scholarship. Vol. XVII, No.4.*

Fine, S. B; (1991). Resilience and human adaptability: who rises above adversity? *American Journal of Occupational Therapy.* Jun;45(6):493-503. Review.

Fine, S.B. (1991), Resiliency and human adaptability: who rises above adversity? 1990 Eleanor Clarke Slagle Lecture. *American Journal of Occupational Therapy*, Jun;45_(6) 493503. Review.

Fink, S.V. (1995, May-June). The influences of family resources and family demands on the strains and well-being of caregiving families. *Nurs Res.* 44(3), 139-146.

Foe, EB., Steketee, G. & Olasov, BR., (1989). Behavorial/cognitive conceptualizations of posttraumatic street disorder. *Behavior Therapy* (20), pp.155-176.

Forster, P. (1992), Nature and treatment of acute stress reactions. Austin, L.S., ed. *Responding to disaster: a guide for mental health professionals.* Washington DC: American Psychiatric Press, pp.25-51.

Freud, S. (1959). Formulations on the two principles of mental functioning. In J. Strachey (Ed. And Trans., *Complete psychological works.* Standard edition (Vol. 12). London: Hogarth Press. (Original work published 1911).

Flannery, Raymond, (1986). Personal control, as a moderator variable of life stress: Preliminary inquiry. *Psychological reports*, 58, (pp200-220).

Giller, E.L., Perry, B.D., Southwick, S., & Mason, J.W.(1990). Psychoneuroendocrinology of post-traumatic stress disorder. In M.E. Wolf & A.D. Mosnaim (Eds.), *Post-traumatic Stress Disorder: Etiology, Phenomenology and Treatment.* (pp. 158-170). Washington, D.C. American Psychiatric Press, Inc.

Golden, Thomas, (1991), Swallowed by a snake: The gift of the Masculine side of healing. Maryland.

Goldfeld, A.E., Mollica, R.F., Presavento, BH., & Faraone, S.V. (1988),

The physical and psychological sequalae of torture: Symptomology and diagnosis. *Journal of the American Medical Association.* 259, 2725-2729.

Goldstein, D.S. (1995). *Stress, Catecholamines and Cardiovascular Disease.* New York: Oxford University Press.

Gottesman, D; Lewis, arc; (1982). Differences in crisis reactions among Cancer and surgery patients. *Journal of Consulting and clinical Psychology.* Vol. 50, No. 3 381-388.

Hamilton, I., McCubbin, M., McCubbin, A., Thompson, S. & Allen, C., (1997). *Families Under Stress: What Makes Them Resilient.* American Association of Family and Consumer Sciences Commemorative Lecture. Wahington, D.C.

Herman, J.L., (1992), Trauma and Recovery. New York: Basic Books.

Horowitz, M.J. (1986). Stress-response syndromes: A review of postraumatic and adjustment disorders. *Hospital and Community Psychiatry*, 37(3), 241-249.

Harvey, Mary; (1996). An ecological View of Psychological Trauma and Trauma Recovery. *Journal of Traumatic Stress*, vol. 9, No.

Hawley, Dale; DeHaan, Laura; (1996). Toward a definition of family resilience: Integrating life span and family perspectives. *Family Practice* 35:283-298.

Holaday, M; Terrell, D; (1994). Resiliency characteristics and Rorschach variables in children and adolescents with severe burns. *Journal of Burn Care and Rehabilitation,* Sept/Oct.; 15(5):455-60.

Jacelon, C.S; (1997). The Trait and Process of Resilience. *Journal of Advanced Nursing*, Jan:25(l):123-9.

Janet, P. (1925). Psychological Healing, Vols. 1-2. New York Macmillan, (Original Publication: *Les Medications Psychologiques,* vol. 1-3, Paris, Felix, Alcan, 1919).

Kadner, K.D; (1989). Resilience. Responding to Adversity. *Journal of Psychosocial Mental Health,* Jul:27(7):20-5.

Kadner, K.D., (1989) Resilience. Responding to Adversity. *Journal of Psychosocial Nursing Mental Health,* Jul;27(7):20-5.

Kardiner, A. (1941). *The Traumatic neurosis of war*. New York: Hoeber.

Kellerman, Dana, (1975), The International Webster New Encyclopedic Dictionary, *The English Language Institute of America.* Chicago, Illinois.

Kvale, Steiner,(1996), *Interviews: An Introduction to Qualitative Research Interviewing.* Sage Publications, Newbury Park, CA.

Kinston, W., Rosser, R., (1974), Disaster:effects on mental and physical state. *Journal of Psychosomatic Research,*(18), pp-437-456.

Kiser, L; Ostoja, E; Pruitt, D; (1998). Dealing with stress and trauma in families. *Child and Adolescent Psychiatric Clinics of North America,* 7 (1):87-10

Kolb, Brian, Wishaw, Ian, (1987), *Introduction to brain and behavior.* W.H. Freeman and Company Publishers.

Koller, Patricia Ann, (1992). Family Needs and Coping Strategies During Illness Crisis. *American Association of Clinical Nursing.*

Kosciulek, J; (1997). Relationship of family schema to family adaptation. *Brain Injury, vol. 11 No. 11, 821-830.*

Kubler-Ross, Elizabeth, (1991,) *On Death and Dying*, MacMillan Publishing, New York, N.Y.

Laub, D., & Auerhahn, N.C. (1993), Knowing and not knowing massive psychic trauma: Forms of *Traumatic Memory. international Journal of Psychoanalysis*, 74, pp.287301.

L.T., & Keane, T.M. (1989). Information processing in anxiety disorders: Application to the understanding of post-traumatic stress disorder. *Clinical Psychology Review, 9,* pp. 243-257.

Lindemann, E., (1944), Symptomatology and management of acute grief. *American Psychiatry.* 133:302-6.

LeDoux, J.E. (1992). Emotion as memory: Anatomical systems underlying indelible neural traces. In S-A Christianson (Ed.), *Handbook of emotion and memory* 269-288). Hillside, N.J.:Lawrence Erlbaum.

LeDoux, J.E., Romanski, L., Xagorais, A., (1991), Indelibility of subcortical emotional memories. *Journal.Coqnitive Neuroscience (1),* pp238-243.

Lambert, Clinton; (1999). Psychological Hardiness: State of the Science. *Holistic Nursing Practice,* 13 (3):11-9 Apr.

Lazerus, R. S; (1993). Coping theory and research; past, present and future. *Psychosomatic Medicine*, May-June:55(3):234-47

Leske, J; Jiricka, M; (1998). Impact of family demands and family strengths and capabilities on family well being and adaptation after critical injury. *American Journal Of Critical Care,* Vol. 7, No. 3 pp. 383392.

Lewis, M; Gottesman, D; and Gutstein, S; (1979). The Course and Duration of Crisis. *Journal of Consulting and Clinical Psychology.* Vol. 47, NO. 1, 128-134.

Lindsey, E;and Hills, M; (1992). An Analysis of the Concept of Hardiness. *The Canadian Journal of Nursing Research.* Spring 24(l), 39-50.

Locke, L., Spiraduso, W., Silverman, S., (1993). Proposals That Work. *Sage Publications*:Newbury Park, CA.

Luthar, S; (1993). Annotation: methodologicaland conceptual issues in research on childhood resilience, *Journal of Child Psychology and Psychiatry.* May: 34(4):441-53

Luthar, S; and Zigler, E; (1991). Vulnerability and Competence: A Review of Research on Resilience in Childhood. *Amercan Journal of Orthopsychiatry*, 6 (1), Jan.

McCann, J.L., & Pearlman, L.A. (1990). Psychological trauma and the adult survivor: *Theory, therapy and transformation*. New York:Brunner/Mazel.

Mcfarlane, AC. (1989)The etiology of post-traumatic morbidity: predisposing, precipitating and perpetuating factors. *British Journal Psychiatry* 154:221-228.

McFarlane, AC., (1988), The longitudinal course of posttraumatic morbidity:the range of outcomes and their predictors. *Journal of Nervous Disorders* 176:565-572.

McCubbin, H.I., & McCubbin, M.A. (1988). Typologies of resilient families: Emerging roles of social class and ethnicity. *Family Relations* 37:247-254.

McCubbin, M.A., & Thompson, A.I. (1993). Resiliency in families: The role of family schema and appraisal in family adaptation to crisis (pp. 153-177). In T.H. Brubaker (ed.), *Family relations: Challenges for the future*. Newbury Park CA: Sage Publications.

McCubbin, M.A. & McCubbin, H.I. (1993). Family coping with health crisis: The resiliency model of family stress, adjustment, and adaptation (pp. 21-64). In C. Danielson, B. Hamel-Bissell, & P. Winstead-Fry (eds.), *Families, health, and illness*. St. Louis MO:C.V. Mosby.

Medalie, J; (1985). Stress, Social Support, Coping, and Adjustment. *The Journal of Family Practice*, vol. 20, No. 6: 533-535.

Messner, Edward (1993) *Resilience Enhancement for the Resident Physician.* Harvard University Press. Cambridge, MA.

Miles, M.B. & Huberman, A.M. (1994). *Qualitative Data Analysis.* Thousand Oaks, CA: Sage.

Mirr, M., & Snyder, M. (1995), *Advanced Practice Nursing:A Guide To Professional Development.* Springer Publishing, Minneapolis, Minnesota.

Montgomery, R.J.V., Gonyea, J.G., Hooyman, N.R., (1985) Caregiving and the Experience of Subjective and Objective Burden. *Family Relations*, Vol. 34, 19-26

Nagy, L.M., Morgan, C.A., Southwick, S.M., Charney, D.S. (1993). Open prospective trial of fluoxetine for post traumatic stress disorder. *Journal of Clinical Psychopharmacology*, 13, pp. 107-114.

Nolan, M; Cupples, S; Brown, M; Pierce, L; Lepley, D; Ohler, L. (1992). Perceived stress and coping strategies among families of cardiac transplant candidates during organ waiting period. *Heart Lung*, Nov. -Dec.:21(6):540-7.

Oe, K. (1997). *A Healing Family.* Tokyo:Kodansha International Ltd.

O'Grady, D; Metz, J; (1986). Resilience in Children at high risk for psychological Disorders. *Journal of Pediatric Psychology*, 12 (1):323.

Patterson, J; (1995). *Promoting Resilience in Families Experiencing Stress.* Pediatric Clinic of North America, Feb:42(1):47-63.

Perry, B., Southwick S. and Giller E: Adrenergic receptor regulation in Post-traumaticstressdisorders, *Advances in psychiatry:biological assessment and treatment of post-*

traumatic stress disorder, E. Giller, Editor. 1990, American Psychiatric Press: Washington, D.C.

Perry, Bruce, (1999), *Memories of Fear, Splintered Reflections: Images of the Body in Trauma*, Basic Books.

Perry, Bruce, Pollard, R., Blakely, T., Baker, W., Vigilante, D., (1996), Childhood trauma, the neurobiology of adaptation and use-dependent development of the brain: How states become traits, *Infant Mental Health Journal*, Houston, TX.

Pilisuk, Marc; Parks, Susan, (1988) Caregiving: Where Families Need Help. *Social Work*, Vol. 33, Number 5, Sept.Oct.

Pilisuk, Marc; Wong, Angela, (2001) Social Network Assessment. *Encyclopedia of Psychological Assessment.*

Pollack, D; (1972). Consistency in Crisis and Responses. *Psychological Reports*, Vol. 31, (3):691-693 Dec.

Polk, L; (1997). Toward a Middle Range Theory of Resilience. *Ans Advanced Nursing. Science,* Mar: 19(3):1-13.

Raphael, B., (1986). *When disaster strikes: How individuals and communities cope with catastrophe.* New York:Basic Books.

Rauch, S., Van der Kolk, B.A., Fisler, R., Orr, S.P., Alpert, N.M., Savage, C.R., Fischman, A.J., Jenike, M.A., & Pitman, R.K. (1994, November). *Pet imagery:positron immision scans of traumatic imagery in PTSD patients.* Paper presented at the annual conference of ISTSS

Reagan, Nancy (1999), *I Love You Ronnie, The Letters of Ronald Reagan To Nancy Reagan*, Random House, New York.

Reid, John, (1990), A role for prospective longitudinal investigations in the study of traumatic stress and disasters, *Journal of Applied Psychology,* Oregon Social Learning Center.

Random House Webster's Dictionary. (1993). New York:Ballantine Reference Library.

Reader, J. (1991). Family Perception: a key to Intervention. *AACN Clinical Issues In Critical Care Nursing* (2):188-94 May.

Rhoades, D., Mcfarland, K., (1999). Caregiver Meaning: a Study of Caregivers of Individuals With Mental Illness. *Health Social Work* Nov;24(4):291-8.

Richards, Ruth (1999). Affective Disorders. *Encyclopedia of Creativity.* (Vol. 1), Academic Press.

Rutter, Michael, (1993). Resilience: Some Conceptual Considerations.
Journal of Adolescent Health. Vol. 14(8):526-31

Rutter, M. (1979). Protective Factors in Children's Responses to Stress and Disadvantage. *Primary Prevention of Psychology,* Vol 3 University Press of New England. pp 49-74.

Schacter. D.L. Understanding implicit memory:a cognitive neuroscience approach. *American Psychologist.* 1992, 47, 559-569.

Seelbach, Wayne, (1977). Gender Differences in Expectations for Filial Responsibility. *The Gerentologist* Vol.17, No. 5,

Seigel, Bernie, (1986) *Love, Medicine and Miracles.* Harper & Row, New Haven Ct.

Solomon, SD, Smith, EM, Robins, LN, Fischbach, RL. (1987), Social involvement as a mediator of disaster-induced stress. *Journal of Applied social Psychology* (17) pp.1092-1112.

Seyle, H., (1978). *The Stress of Life*, (2nd ed.). New York: McGraw-Hill

Seligman, M; (1990) *Learned Optimism*. New York: Random House.

Silva, M; (1987). Needs of Spouses of Surgical Patients: a conceptus. *Scholarly Inquiry*, Vol. l(l):29-44. Spring.

Stamm, Beth, (1999) *Secondary Traumatic Stress. Self-care Issues for Clinicians, Researchers and Educators*. Lutherville, MD., Sidran Press.

Stone, Arthur; (1983). Assessment of Coping Efficacy: A Comment. *Journal of Behavioral Medicine*, Vol. 8, No. 2.

Twibell, R; (1998). Family Coping During Critical Illness, *Dimensions of Critical Care Nursing*, Vol. 17, (2):100-112 Mar-Apr.

Ursano, Robert; (1995). Post-Traumatic Stress Disorder: Psychiatric Responses to Trauma and Disaster, *Harvard Review Psychiatry.*, 3:196-209.

Ursano, RJ, McCarrol, JE, (1990), The nature of the traumatic stressor:handling dead bodies. *Journal of Nervous Mental Disorders.* (178), pp.396-398.

Ursano, Robert, Holloway, H.C., (1985), Military Psychiatry. In Kaplan HI, Sadock, B.J., (Eds.). *Comprehensive textbook of psychiatry. (4 th ed., pp. 1900*-9) Baltimore: Williams & Wilkins .

Ursano, R.J., McCaughy, B.C., Fullerton, C.S. (1994), The structure of human chaos. In: Ursano, R.J. McCaughy BG, Fullerton CS, (Eds.), *Individual and community responses to trauma and disaster:the structure of human chaos.* London:Cambridge University Press, pp.3-27

Ursano, RJ, Fullerton, CS, Wright, Km, McCarroll, JE, Norwood, AK, Dineen, MM, (1992), *Disaster workers: trauma and social support.* Bethesda, Maryland:Uniformed Services University of the Health Sciences, DTIC_publication no ADB 165599.

Valent, Paul, (1998), Introduction to Survival Strategies, *Survival to fulfillment: a framework for the lifetrauma dialectic.*(pp.115-123). Philadelphia: Brunner/Mazel.

Van der Hart, 0., Steele, K., Boon, S., & Brown, P.(1993), The treatment of traumatic memories: Synthesis, realization, and integration. *Dissociation, 6,_*(pp.162-180).

Van der Kolk, B.A., Roth, S., Pelcovitz, D. & Mandel F. (1993)Complex PTSD: Results of the PTSD trials for DSM IV; *American Psychiatric Association.*

Van der Kolk, B.A. (1994). The body keeps the score:Memory and the evolving psychobiology of posttraumatic stress. *Harvard Review Psychiatry.*

Van der Kolk, B. & Fisler, Rita, (1995), *Dissociation and the Fragmentary Nature of Traumatic Memories*, Harvard Medical School Department of Psychiatry_.

Van der Kolk, B.A. & Fisler, R. (1994). Childhood abuse neglect and loss of self-regulation. *Bulletin of Menninger Clinic, 58,_*145-168.

Van der Kolk, B.A., & van der Hart, 0. (1991). The intrusive past: The flexibility of memory and the engraving of trauma. *American Imago, 48_(4)*, 425-454.

Van der Kolk, B.A., & Saporta, J., (1991), The biological response to psychic trauma:mechanisms and treatment of intrusion and numbing. *Anxiety Research (4)* 199-212.

Van Der Kolk, B., Pelcovitz, D., Roth, S., Mandel, F., McFarlane, A., Herman, J., (1996), Dissociation, Somatization, Affect Dysregulation: The Complexity of Adaption to Trauma. *American Journal of Psychiatry.* 153:7, July Festchrift Supplement.

Walsh, Froma; (1996). The Concept of Famly Resilience: Crisis and Challenge. *Family Process, Vol. 35, No. 3:* 261-281.

Websters Dictionary New College (1993), New York: Ballantine Reference Library.

Wills, T.A. & Shinar, O. (2000). Measuring perceived and received social support. In S. Cohen, L. G. Underwood & B. H. Gottleib. *Social Support Measurement and Intervention: A Guide for Health and Social Scientists.* Oxford:Oxford University Press, 86-135.

Weiss, R.S. (1994). *Learning from Strangers: The art and method of qualitative interview studies.* New York: Free Press.

Weiss, R; (1988). Is It Possible To Prepare For Trauma? *Journal of Palliative Care, Vol. 4, (1-2):* pp.74-6 May.

Wollen, S. & Wollen, S. (1993), *The Resilient Self, How survivors of troubled families rise above adversity.* Villard Books; Random House, N.Y

Wolff, S; (1995). The Concept of Resilience. *Australian and New Zealand Journal of Psychiatry. 29 (4)*: pp.565-74 Dec.

Wyman, P; Cowen, E; Work, W; and Parker, G; (1991). Developmental and Family Milieu Correlates of Resilience in Urban Children Who Have Experienced Major Life Stress. *American Journal of Community Psychology, Vol. 19, No.*

Yehuda, R., Schmeidler, J., Elkin, A., Houshmand, B., Seiver, L., Binder-byrnes, K., Wainberg, M., Aferiot, D., Lehman, A., Song GuoL., Kwei Yang, Ren, (1997), Phenomenology and psychobiology of the intergenerational response to trauma, *Intergenerational Handbook of Multigenerational Legacies of Trauma*

APPENDIX B

<u>Participant Information Questionnaire</u>

Code #________________

Presenter______________

Please fill out the information below. Leave blank any questions that you don't wish to respond to. Thank you for your participation in this study.

Date______________

Name____

Address____

Telephone____

E-Mail______________

Gender ( ) Male ( ) Female

Education______________ Highest Degree__________________________

Age ________________ Occupation __________________________

Ethnic Background: ( ) Caucasian ( ) Afro-American ( ) Native American ( ) Asian ( ) Other:______________

Income Level ( ) 15,000-25,000, ( )25,000-50,000,( )50,000-100,000, ( ) 100,000-500,000

Have you ever seen a therapist? ( ) yes, ( ) no

APPENDIX D

<u>Specific Questions for Semi-Structured Qualitative Interview</u>

<u>(Cooney, 2002)</u>

(1) What inspired or led you to become a caregiver: was it by choice or duty?

(2) How has this positively or negatively impacted your life?

(3) Did you have doubts about your ability or willingness to take on this role?

(4) What do you perceive to be the most important qualities for adaptation and endurance?

(5) In retrospect, would you do differently to balance the care for the patient and the care for yourself?

(6) Has your ability to interact with other relationships or social connectedness been impacted by this caregiving experience?

(7) How do you feel this experience has impacted your ability to enjoy and progress in other areas of your life?

(8) Have hope and spirituality been factors in your ability to cope and endure throughout this experience?

APPENDIX F

Six Qualitative Self-Report Questions (Cooney, 2002)

1. What inspired or challenged you to become a caregiver?

____

____

2. What are the qualities that have enabled you to adapt, endure and

    maintain your sense of resiliency?

____

____

3. How has caregiving positively affected your life?

____

____

4. How has caregiving negatively affected your life.

____

____

4. What surprising thing have you learned about yourself from this experience?

____

____

5. What coping mechanisms would you recommend to other caregivers?

____

____

Susan Cooney, Ph.D.

About the Author

Dr. Cooney has Ph.D. in clinical psychology and lives in a suburb of Boston. She has a decade of experience with acute psychiatric patients in the Emergency/Trauma Department at Massachusetts General Hospital. Her work with acute psychiatric issues and pathology as well as work with the families following the events of 9/11 in New York has exposed her to a wide array of responses to stress and grief. This knowledge has inspired her to delve further into this arena.